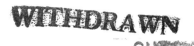

Getting into

Nursing & Midwifery Courses

Getting into guides

Getting into

Nursing & Midwifery Courses

Wendy Reed

trotman t

Getting into Nursing & Midwifery Courses

This 1st edition published in 2013 by Trotman Publishing, an imprint of Crimson Publishing Limited, Westminster House, Kew Road, Richmond, Surrey TW9 2ND

© Trotman Publishing 2013

Author: Wendy Reed

British Library Cataloguing in Publication Data
A catalogue record for this book is available from the British Library

ISBN 978 1 906041 96 0

Typeset by IDSUK (DataConnection) Ltd
Printed and bound in the UK by TJ International Ltd, Padstow, Cornwall

Contents

About the author

Wendy Reed is a professionally trained careers adviser who has worked in schools, with further and higher education students, graduates and adults, and is now a freelance careers writer. She is the author of *Working in Hospitals*, *Working in Social Care* and *Working in Education* and has written articles and content for careers websites including the Prospects graduate careers website. She has many years' experience of helping both A level students and Access to Higher Education students make applications to UCAS, including to nursing and midwifery courses, and to write personal statements.

Acknowledgements

I would like to thank the university admissions tutors and students who gave up their time to answer my many questions, share their experiences and provide valuable contributions that helped inform the content of the book.

Particular thanks go to Heather Bower, Lead Midwife for Education and Sally Morey, admissions tutor for adult nursing at Oxford Brookes University who found time to speak to me at one of the busiest times of the application cycle. I would also like to extend thanks to Luisa Acosta and Ramona Minette, admissions tutors at the University of West London. Also to Jane Alexander at Reading College who put me in contact with former Access to Higher Education students, to give me an insight into the mature-student route into nursing and midwifery.

Thanks also go to Caroline Farrar and the nursing students of De Montfort University, both current and recently qualified: Jessica Potter, Charlotte Hings, Holly Janine Bexson Smith, Ros Dampier, Holly Southall and Sarah Collin amongst others . . . for agreeing to be interviewed and providing an excellent insight for prospective students into studying nursing and career options beyond.

Introduction

This book is a new addition to the series of 'Getting into' titles as a response to the increased popularity of nursing and midwifery courses and to provide guidance on making the best possible application to maximise your chances of securing a place.

How popular are nursing and midwifery courses?

The number of applications to nursing courses has risen rapidly over the last few years and remains high. This has come at the same time as a decrease in the number of available places. According to UCAS, in 2010 there were 194,214 applications and 27,079 acceptances on to courses, a ratio of 7.2 applications to each place; in 2011 there were 218,599 applications and 24,587 acceptances on to courses, a ratio of 8.9 applications to each place over all nursing courses. In 2012 there were 212,572 applications and 23,836 acceptances, again a ratio of 8.9 applications to each place. On more popular courses the ratio can be much higher. The University of Birmingham, for example, had 1,282 applications for 104 places on their undergraduate nursing degree.

Midwifery has been popular for a while and over the last few years applications have been on a steady upward trend: the number of applicants to each place is now at least 20:1. In 2012 Oxford Brookes University had over 600 applicants for 28 places. There has been a slight increase in the number of places on courses but the number of applicants has also increased.

How this book can help

In order to stand a chance of securing a place, it is really important to make a good application, including a first-rate personal statement, and to be fully prepared for selection days and interviews. The key to making a good application, according to admissions tutors for both nursing and midwifery, is to demonstrate that you have a full understanding of what the role of a nurse or midwife involves in today's health service and that you have fully considered whether you have the values, personal attributes and skills to make an effective nurse or midwife. This book will take you through the steps needed to fully demonstrate that you have done the preparation needed to make this decision. This includes helping you choose the right branch of nursing for you, selecting the most appropriate course, finding relevant work experience, making an effective application and personal statement, and performing well at selection days. You will be helped along by case studies and insider tips and advice from university admissions tutors, current students and newly qualified nurses or midwives.

Choosing your branch of nursing

Before applying to study nursing, in most cases you have to make a choice of which branch of nursing to study. This book has a particular focus on the importance of making the correct choice for you, with practical considerations to take into account as well as personal preference. There are generally more places on courses for adult nursing and some universities offer both an autumn and a spring start. There are fewer places for midwifery but some courses have both autumn and spring starts. Overall there are fewer places for mental health, learning disability and children's nursing but this can vary greatly from area to area. Children's nursing is very popular with a small number of places to numbers of applications received. In 2012 at Swansea University, for example, there were 300 applicants for 15 places.

Entry requirements on the increase

From September 2013 anyone wanting to train as a nurse will need to study a degree course and must meet the entry requirements for study at degree level. In general, universities have raised the entry requirements for nursing and midwifery degree courses, in part due to the changing demands of the job but also due to the high demand for places. This book will cover the new entry requirements, including numeracy, literacy and grade requirements, and advice for a range of applicants, including mature students.

About this book

Chapter 1 introduces to you what nurses and midwives do, how nursing and midwifery have changed in recent years and current employment prospects. The chapter concludes with information on the Nursing and Midwifery Council (NMC), the professional body representing UK nurses and midwives, its purpose and the importance of the code of professional standards for nurses and midwives.

The range of available qualifications, depending on your entry level, and the specific areas of nursing and midwifery that might suit you are important considerations when joining either profession: **Chapter 2** deals with the many choices available. We will look at the structure of courses, including the range of practical placements you can expect in each branch of nursing and in midwifery.

Relevant work experience is a vital requirement for applying to nursing and midwifery courses. In **Chapter 3** we will look at what universities want in terms of experience and how you can go about finding this. We will look at the types of work experience useful for each branch of nursing and how to present this in an effective personal statement.

In **Chapter 4** we will look at factors important in choosing your course; entry requirements and how they differ from course to course; choosing a university; and the skills needed for each branch of nursing and for midwifery.

Chapter 5 takes you through how to apply using the online UCAS application in step-by-step detail, with a focus on the importance of an early application and suggested timetables to enable this to happen. We will also look at how to deal with unsuccessful applications.

In **Chapter 6** we focus on one of the most important parts of your UCAS application – the personal statement. You will find detailed information about suggested content and structure with tips from the people who will read them – admissions tutors.

Chapter 7 gives detailed information about what to expect at a selection day and how to prepare for individual interviews, group interviews and other selection activities.

Much of the course information you will find on university websites deals with standard entry requirements for A level students. **Chapter 8** gives guidance to other applicants, mature students, EU or international students, those with a disability or those who have additional needs.

A level results day is the topic of **Chapter 9**. This chapter includes advice on how to prepare for receiving your results and deals with the situations you might find yourself in and how you should react, including what to do if you miss a grade or if you are unsuccessful in getting a place and want to reapply.

Chapter 10 deals with fees and funding and gives details of the NHS bursary, how to apply and other sources of funding you may be eligible for.

Careers in nursing and midwifery are covered in **Chapter 11**. We look at each branch of nursing and midwifery, what it can involve, where you can work and the specialist areas into which you can move. This chapter also covers what you can expect to be paid and the opportunities available for progression into teaching, research and management opportunities. The focus of the chapter is not a complete guide to all career opportunities but to help you decide which branch of nursing is for you or whether to study midwifery, based on the scope for career opportunities. We also look at working abroad and armed-forces nursing.

Chapter 12 gives contact details and websites for useful organisations, journals, careers information, funding and other useful sources of information on nursing and midwifery.

Finally, we have included a **glossary** of some medical terms and other phrases related to studying nursing and midwifery. Having knowledge of the correct terminology shows you have done some background reading and signals a better understanding of your chosen subject area, which will help your application stand out from that of the crowd.

The information in this book was correct at the time of writing. Please be aware that higher education courses, entry requirements and funding are all subject to change and you should check the websites provided for updates before making an application.

By the end of the book, you should have gained the confidence to make an informed, effective and hopefully successful application to nursing or midwifery.

1 | Is nursing or midwifery for me?

Choosing to study nursing or midwifery is a challenging yet reward-ing career choice and one where you can make a positive contribu-tion to improving people's lives. Nurses and midwives are vital profes-sionals in the front-line health team and their roles have evolved to take on more responsibility and to work more independently. Jobs have also become more varied with nurses and midwives working not just in tra-ditional hospital settings but also in the community, in GP surgeries and health clinics, residential homes, private healthcare, schools, prisons, the armed forces, for charities, such as Macmillan Cancer Support, and overseas in developing countries.

This chapter will cover employment prospects for nurses and midwives, an introduction to what they do and how their roles are changing. It will also look at the importance of the Nursing and Midwifery Council (NMC) and the professional code of conduct for nurses and midwives.

What are the employment prospects?

In October 2012 there were 633,477 nurses and 41,174 midwives on the NMC register. More than 1 in 10 nurses are men and there are 162 male midwives; these numbers are slowly increasing.

You may be concerned about the effect the current recession has had on healthcare spending, the reorganisation of the NHS and the resulting impact this has had on nursing and midwifery. Although there has been a reduction in the number of healthcare jobs, these have been mostly in administrative and managerial roles, with a government pledge to pro-tect spending on front-line jobs such as nursing and midwifery. Some Healthcare Trusts are making savings in other ways to avoid cutting posts. However, overall there has been a decrease in the number of nursing posts but a slight increase in those for midwives.

According to the *Nursing Times*, in the last 12 months the number of qual-ified nurses working in the sector has fallen by 0.6%. Figures for public-health nursing and midwifery are better with the number of midwives up by 438, health visitors up by 298 and school nurses up by 22. These figures don't include nurses working in the private sector, local authorities and new social enterprises (*Nursing Times* September 2012).

In fact some changes to the structure of the healthcare system may have an indirect positive impact on working as a nurse or midwife. Although some hospital departments have been closed, this has been in favour of creating fewer, better-staffed and better-equipped units at larger hospitals and there are plans to increase the use of technology to allow nurses to spend less time on paperwork and more time 'at the bedside'. There are moves to provide more care outside hospitals in the community, 24-hour care and more services for the elderly (a growing part of the population), therefore more opportunity for community nursing.

> *The role will continue to develop, and change has always been part of nursing. The future is exciting for nursing with many more specialist and autonomous roles and it is more diverse than it used to be although, as always, with patients at the centre. Nurses can care for patients in many different settings, with many more roles now based in the community. A lot of care settings that wouldn't originally take newly registered nurses now do, including for example intensive care and district nursing. Healthcare Trusts are using different ways to make savings and may not necessarily cut the number of nursing jobs. Potential students should check the employment rates for the university courses they are interested in applying to.*
>
> Sally Morey, admissions tutor for adult nursing at
> Oxford Brookes University

What do nurses and midwives do?

Nurses

Nurses work with people from a range of ages with both physical and mental-health conditions, using both caring and counselling skills. These include people who are unwell or recovering from accidents, as well as those who have healthcare needs due to age or disability. Nurses help people to live more comfortable and independent lives, or to have a peaceful end to life. They also have a role to promote good health through education.

Nurses work in many different settings and their roles vary enormously. When deciding to become a nurse, from the outset you have to choose one of the following four 'branches' of nursing to train in: adult, children's, mental health, or learning disability.

Adult

Adult nurses work with a wide range of people from young adults to the elderly with both long-term and short-term health conditions. They work in hospital wards or clinics and increasingly in the community.

Children's

This branch of nursing involves learning to work with children of all ages, from babies to teenagers, and with a child's family or carers to minimise the effects health problems can have on a child's development.

Mental health

Mental-health nurses support people who have a range of mental-health problems from anxiety and depression to personality or psychological disorders. The job focuses on promoting recovery or helping clients come to terms with illness and leading a positive life.

Learning disability

Nurses who choose this branch of nursing provide specialist healthcare, in partnership with families and carers, for people with a wide range of physical and mental-health conditions. Learning-disability nurses support people to integrate into society by helping them lead a more independent and healthy life.

See Chapter 11 for further information on the careers to which these different branches can lead.

Midwives

Midwives provide professional advice, care and support for women, their partners and families before, during and after the birth of a child. They work in multi-professional teams in hospitals and, in recent years, increasingly in people's homes and the community.

> **TIP!**
>
> Don't go into midwifery if you only want to work with babies – increasingly the main focus of the role is to support the mother during pregnancy, labour and childbirth.

See Chapter 11 for further information on the careers open to midwives.

> *Maternity care assistants are increasingly being given more responsibility for the post-natal care period. A midwife may only see a woman a few times after the birth and further home visits and care are provided by the maternity care assistant. This is an unfortunate erosion of the midwife's role and in the future I would predict that midwives will focus more on antenatal care, labour and birth.*
>
> Heather Bower, Lead Midwife for Education at
> Oxford Brookes University

Nursing and midwifery today

Practice and training in nursing and midwifery have changed and developed dramatically over the last 20 years. That is not to say that everything has changed. Patients still have the same problems as patients of 100 years ago – pain, discomfort, loss of independence – and nurses and midwives continue to need the same listening and caring skills to treat and support them. However, the way in which nurses and midwives work has changed radically, as have their responsibilities, job titles and employers. Much of this change has come about with increased professionalism, technical advances in healthcare and improved training.

Improvements in career-progression routes for nurses and midwives mean that they can more easily take on management responsibilities or move into specialist areas such as occupational-health nursing, practice nursing, theatre nursing or neonatal nursing (working with newborn babies who are sick or born prematurely). There are opportunities for both nurses and midwives to progress to a consultant role, combining practice with being a leader for improvements in healthcare practice, or to an education role to train student nurses and midwives. With the trend for community-based care and focus on preventive treatment in the home, nurses and midwives are increasingly working in the community and promoting healthy living. They are also working for a wider range of employers, including charities, and in private healthcare. See Chapter 11 for more on career progression.

> *Students should think outside of just acute hospital roles, more and more care is out in the community and can be in specialist roles such as asthma nurse or diabetes nurse.*
>
> Admissions tutor for nursing

Nursing and Midwifery Council

To practise as a nurse you need to be professionally registered with the Nursing and Midwifery Council (NMC), the regulatory body that ensures that all nurses are properly trained and fit to perform their job. If you wish to train to be a nurse or a midwife, you need to complete an NMC-approved course and then register with the NMC. Formal registration and recognition in nursing and midwifery are far from new. The UK register of midwives was established in 1902 and nurse registration in 1919.

So what does the NMC do?

The primary purpose of the NMC is to safeguard the health and well-being of the public. This includes:

- registration of all nurses and midwives in the UK to ensure that they are properly qualified and can do their job competently
- setting the standards of education, training and performance so that nurses and midwives can deliver high-quality healthcare consistently throughout their careers
- ensuring that nurses and midwives keep their skills and knowledge up to date and uphold professional standards
- using fair processes to investigate allegations made against nurses and midwives who may not have followed the code of professional standards.

Changes to the NMC

The NMC is focusing more on its primary role as a regulator and will no longer offer an email and phone advice service for nurses and midwives, but it is working to improve the advice section of its website. It is developing a revalidation process to ensure that nurses and midwives remain fit to practise throughout their careers and it is also revising the rules and standards for midwives.

Why is the code of professional standards important?

Nurses and midwives have a very responsible job. They need to be accountable: that is, to take responsibility for their actions, know their limitations and not do more than their experience or training allows. They also need to be responsible with personal information, for example, confidential patient records. They are expected to use professional knowledge to problem-solve, identify solutions and make independent decisions and, as the most frequent point of contact for patients, answer questions from patients and families.

What skills and qualities do I need as a nurse or midwife?

Communication

You need to enjoy and be good at listening and communicating with a wide range of people.

Teamwork

Healthcare workers increasingly work in multidisciplinary teams. You need to like the idea of working in a team with the shared aim to care for patients.

Emotional maturity

Nurses and midwives need to stay calm in stressful situations, be alert to changes in patient conditions and react quickly and efficiently in an emergency.

If you feel that working in nursing or midwifery may be for you and that you have the right skills and enthusiasm, then read on to find out more about study routes and how you can maximise your chances of getting onto a nursing or midwifery degree.

2 | Studying nursing and midwifery

In this chapter we will look at the range of qualifications available to become a nurse or midwife, how the courses are structured and teaching styles used. This will include degree, graduate diploma and master's level pre-registration courses. Comments from current students will illustrate some of the demands of studying nursing, both academic and practical. We will also look in more detail at the different branches of nursing and at midwifery courses to help you begin to consider which direction is right for you. Student experiences of being on placement will help inform you how these branches can differ.

> It is important to remember that to work as a nurse or midwife in the UK you must be registered with the NMC. This means successfully completing a degree course approved by the NMC. Use the UCAS course search for a list of pre-registration degree, graduate diploma and master's level courses. You can also use www. nmc-uk.org/Approved-Programmes for both pre-registration and post-registration NMC-approved courses.

The chapter concludes with information on access to nursing courses designed specifically for mature students who do not yet have the qualifications to apply directly for a degree and need further study to reach this level.

Nursing courses

Courses are titled Bachelor of Science (BSc) or Bachelor of Nursing (BN or BNurs) and usually lead to a student being qualified in a specialist branch of nursing. Approved courses generally take three or four years full-time, although some are available part-time and may be aimed at those already working in the healthcare sector who wish to progress to a degree. Courses are 50% university education and 50% healthcare placements.

Placements are an important part of nurse training as they give you the chance to put the theory and skills you have learnt on the course into practice. They can include gaining experience in a variety of hospital wards and in community health. Some courses offer the opportunity to carry out an elective placement (a placement of your choice), possibly overseas. We will look at placements in more detail further on in the chapter (see page 16).

Choosing your branch of nursing

In most cases before you apply you have to choose between four specialist branches of nursing:

- adult
- children's
- mental health
- learning disability.

Each year universities are instructed by their local Healthcare Trust as to how many places they can offer for each branch of nursing. This is because the health service works with universities to forward-plan its workforce needs – in essence it calculates and plans for specific num-bers of nurses and midwives to qualify three or four years ahead of when they are required.

There are generally more places on adult-nursing courses, with smaller numbers of places on the other three branches. Generally children's nursing is very popular with more applicants to each place. Contact universities to find out how many places they offer for each branch.

It is very important to spend time considering which branch of nursing is right for you before you apply. As well as information on the structure and content of the different branches further on in this chapter, you may find the information in Chapter 4 on the skills needed for each branch, and in Chapter 11 on careers and specialist nursing roles to which each branch can lead useful to make comparisons. Pages 15–23 look at the typical content of the different branches of nursing courses.

Other types of courses

Dual-registration courses

Several universities offer four-year dual-registration courses, which allow you to qualify and register with the NMC in two chosen branches of nursing, from adult, children's, mental health, and learning disability, in a range of combinations. Although a longer course, you may end up with a wider range of skills, competencies and experiences, which will be attractive to employers. The NMC Approved Programmes course finder, www.nmc-uk.org/Approved-Programmes, is useful to locate dual-registration courses, currently offered at De Montfort University, Oxford Brookes University, and the University of Southampton. Funding through an NHS bursary is available for the entire course but may be pro rata over the four years. See Chapter 10 for more information on funding.

General nursing degree

A small number of universities, such as the University of Birmingham, offer a general nursing degree, where a choice of specialist branch doesn't need to be made until the end of the first year. Although there are benefits to not having to make a choice (you will have the first year of the course to try a range of placements to help with your decision), the University of Birmingham is keen to point out that you must be aware that as there are fewer places on the course for some branches of nursing, such as children's nursing, by opting for this course you take a risk that you may not be able to qualify in your preferred branch.

Decelerated courses

If you need greater flexibility to manage your time, De Montfort University currently offers four-year decelerated courses. The course content is the same as a three-year course but stretched over four years. NHS bursaries are available for the entire course but may be pro rata over the four years. See Chapter 10 for funding information.

Four-year undergraduate master's degree

It is also possible to study a four-year MSci at the University of Nottingham, which is a pre-registration degree followed by one year of master's level postgraduate study. This may be particularly appropriate if you want to combine training to be a nurse with gaining research skills or are interested in nurse education, research or policy making. In the fourth year, students complete a research dissertation. The course allows you to integrate research skills, theory and clinical practice. The course includes an elective placement in the UK or abroad.

Postgraduate diploma courses

Postgraduate diploma (GDN PgDip) nursing courses lasting around two years are available for those wishing to train as a nurse after completing a first degree. You would need an honours degree in a subject relevant to nursing, e.g. biological science, social sciences, psychology, behavioural sciences or health studies. Some courses may consider graduates with other degrees. It is also possible to study courses that combine registration for nursing with an MSc in nursing, such as at Oxford Brookes University. NHS bursaries are also available for these courses.

Health-foundation courses

Four-year nursing or midwifery courses with an initial health-foundation year are aimed at those who do not have the level or subject requirements for a degree: for example, if you did not study a science A level, got lower-than-expected grades in science or were unable to complete your studies due to illness. Entry requirements will be lower than for degree courses, but you will still need two A levels or equivalent at required grades, or equivalent UCAS points. You would also need GCSEs at C in maths and English or equivalent.

The course will be aimed at a wide range of students wishing to progress to health or medical-related degrees and will include core modules and skills relevant to all areas, such as numeracy, IT, communication skills and counselling skills. You will also be able to study academic modules related to your chosen degree programme. The course may include local day placements to give an insight into the roles of different healthcare professionals.

Bear in mind that progression to the degree part of the course will not be guaranteed and may be subject to passing all foundation-year modules at a certain percentage level.

NHS bursaries are available to cover the entire course but may be pro rata over the four years. See Chapter 10 on funding for more information.

Use the UCAS course search at www.ucas.com to locate degree courses with a health-foundation year; applications can be made through UCAS.

Midwifery courses

Courses are mostly direct-entry Bachelor of Science (BSc) or Bachelor of Midwifery (BMid or BM). Midwifery degrees, like nursing degrees, comprise roughly 50% theoretical training and 50% healthcare placements. Competition for places is intense. As with nursing, placements take place in a variety of settings, in hospitals and the community. Most courses last three years.

Postgraduate diplomas in midwifery (GDN PgDip) are available for graduates with relevant degrees, who wish to convert to midwifery.

Oxford Brookes University offers a Midwifery (Pre-registration) MSc for those with relevant biological-science degrees who want a course leading to registration as a midwife combined with gaining a master's degree. This may be particularly attractive to those who wish to consider a future research or teaching career combined with practising as a midwife.

Midwifery short programme

A small number of courses are available for qualified and registered nurses (usually adult nurses) wishing to train as midwives. The course lasts a minimum of 18 months, and involves a similar amount of supervised practice as in a three-year direct-entry course. There is considerable competition for places. The NMC Approved Programmes course finder, www.nmc-uk.org/Approved-Programmes, is useful to locate 18-month programmes.

Regional differences

In Scotland courses are three years long to gain an ordinary level degree (without dissertation) or four years for an honours degree (with dissertation) leading to registration as a nurse or midwife. You choose to study a general course leading to registration as an adult nurse, or a specialist branch leading to children's, mental-health or learning-disability nursing. Courses usually have a two-year foundation followed by two years specialising in a particular branch.

Typical course content

Theoretical learning

The theoretical side of nursing and midwifery courses combines traditional teaching styles, such as lectures and seminars, with small-group tutorials and project work using e-learning. Access to lectures comprising handouts and worksheets online and, in some cases, virtual scenarios to practise nursing procedures is increasingly being offered. Courses also include problem-solving exercises (enquiry-based learning) and case studies.

On many courses teaching is delivered by experienced nurses and nurse consultants as well as by academic staff. Learning is often shared, through multi-professional modules, with other students from related health and social-work courses, to develop interdisciplinary working and teamwork skills and to gain an understanding of wider issues in the sector. You may have blocks of time assigned to personal study, where you will be expected to research and read around topics from lectures and use personal reflection to assess how you are progressing, to prepare you for the continuing professional development (CPD) required of every qualified nurse and midwife. Some courses have more emphasis on research-based study or may encourage students to come up with innovative ideas to challenge traditional nursing practice.

Clinical-simulation suites

Many courses offer the opportunity to acquire practical skills using clinical-simulation suites: university departments set up to mirror hospital, community or home settings. Computerised dummies, called 'sim men', are used to create a realistic experience; these are models that breathe and talk and can simulate conditions such as cardiac arrest or falling blood pressure. The rooms also include equipment such as electric beds, moving and handling equipment and monitoring equipment. This enables the student to practise real-life clinical skills and procedures in safe and supervised conditions.

Placements

You will go out on placement several times during the course, often with a longer placement in the final year as a transition to professional practice. On placement you are expected to work shifts, including weekends and nights, and to work full-time hours in the same way as a qualified nurse or midwife would, to experience the reality of the job. You can usually expect support from a linked-university tutor and a workplace mentor, usually a qualified nurse or midwife.

> *With administering medication and injections I have direct supervision from my mentor, with other areas, such as writing care plans or treatment objectives, I may ask for some help before writing my own plan then have it checked before presenting it at a multidisciplinary meeting.*
>
> Ros Dampier, second-year mental-health nursing student at De Montfort University

Many courses offer an elective placement (a placement of your choice) in the UK or abroad. Bear in mind that you may have to organise and fund placements abroad yourself but universities often offer overseas-exchange programmes and can sometimes help with funding. This could include experiencing nursing in a developing country, gaining an insight into healthcare internationally, or studying at an overseas university.

Assessments

Courses are assessed through coursework – essays, projects, writing professional reports and making presentations, and by exams. Clinical practice is assessed through observed clinical simulations and on placement by the workplace mentor.

The opinions of current students that follow may give you an idea of some of the academic demands of a nursing degree:

> *The most challenging part of the course is processing all the information I amass from lectures and placements and keeping up with independent study. When on placement I only have one study day a week, which includes attending university lectures.*
>
> Charlotte Hings, third-year learning-disability nursing student at De Montfort University

*The hardest thing about the course so far is reading around
a subject after a lecture, finding the time to do the necessary
amount of independent study.*

Holly Janine Bexson Smith, first-year student
at De Montfort University

*What I find most difficult is writing assignments and doing exams,
as I have dyslexia. However, I get a lot of one-to-one support
at university and extra tuition if I need it, such as extra time
for exams. The jump from school to university is quite difficult;
adjusting to self-directed learning and doing all the background
reading required is difficult.*

Jessica Potter, third-year learning-disability nursing
student at De Montfort University

*The most challenging part of my course has been the OSCE
(objective structured clinical examination) practical examinations.
These take place in the simulation suite where you are given a
scenario relating to an individual patient (mannequin), where you
have to make observations, carry out an assessment and then
suggest how you would treat, backing this up with evidence. It is
demanding and requires memorising a lot of information and being
able to apply this theory to practice.*

Victoria Lynne, third-year children's nursing student
at Birmingham City University

*To get through your training to become an adult nurse you need
to be hard-working and willing to put a lot of your personal life on
hold. You don't get long holidays and you can't go out drinking at
the weekends because you will be working most of them!*

Holly Southall, recently qualified adult nurse
from De Montfort University

Structure of courses

In general, all nursing and midwifery courses include:

- academic studies: such as biological sciences and social sciences
- professional studies: the role of a nurse
- developing skills: such as communication, teamwork and leadership
- practical competencies: acquired through simulations and placements.

Courses have a common core first year with a general introduction to
both theory and practice and in the second year introduce study and
practice related to your chosen branch of nursing. In the final year there
is often a research-based dissertation.

In all branches of nursing and midwifery you will spend around 50% of the course based at a university. Courses combine learning background theory and acquiring clinical-care skills and will include topics such as:

- life sciences: development of the human body and mind, anatomy, physiology
- social sciences: healthcare psychology, political, economic and social influences on care
- person-centred care, and care within the context of family and carers
- personal and professional accountability, ethics and legal issues, equality and diversity
- quality and safety in healthcare
- public health and health promotion.

Skills

- clinical-care skills
- transferable skills: communication, advocacy, teamwork.

Managing and leading care

- inter-professional working and shared decision making, collaboration
- advising and educating patients and other professionals
- nursing or midwifery management.

Research skills

- evidence-based care: using up-to-date research to inform care practices
- being innovative and querying care practices in response to patient need.

All branches of nursing include the main topics above. We will now look at the different branches of nursing and how additional topics studied may differ to help you begin to choose the right branch for you.

Adult nursing

The focus of this branch of nursing is to learn to deliver care to clients of all ages from 18 to the elderly. You will learn to care for a wide variety of adults, from all walks of life and in a range of settings, including the community. As well as the general modules listed above, courses can include:

- assessment and planning practices
- acute medical/surgical nursing, A&E and critical care
- nursing long-term conditions
- end-of-life care

- primary healthcare
- community care
- medicine management.

Placements

It is arranged that 50% of the course is spent on a variety of place-ments, organised by your university in partnership with local hospitals and healthcare providers, to gain experience of the breadth of adult-nursing provision in your local area. You will go out on placement throughout the period of the course, usually culminating in a longer placement to act as a transition to starting work as a qualified practitio-ner. Placements can be in:

- hospitals: in a range of departments, including both medical and surgical wards, such as intensive care, accident and emergency, theatre and recovery rooms
- primary care: such as GP surgeries, health centres
- community care: in community treatment centres, nursing homes and hospice care for the elderly, rehabilitation settings with district nurses and in patients' own homes.

Placements may include both NHS and private organisations. You can usually expect to be supervised, mentored and assessed by experi-enced adult nurses.

> By the final placement the level of responsibility will depend on a student's previous experiences and what is appropriate in that care setting. All students have to achieve core competencies at the required level for registration, but if appropriate will take on more; in community nursing, for example, a student may be managing a caseload. They will also have experience of the management aspects of nursing care.
>
> Sally Morey, admissions tutor for adult nursing
> at Oxford Brookes University

Children's nursing

The focus of children's nursing is working with parents to promote the health and well-being of children. The work is interdisciplinary, working with many other professionals. The course often begins with study of the healthy child, progressing to looking at the healthcare needs of sick children before possibly moving into more-specialist areas, such as chil-dren with mental-health issues, learning disabilities or acute illnesses. Courses cover delivering care to newborn babies, to adolescents, and in a range of settings. In addition to the general nursing modules listed earlier in the chapter, courses can include:

- promoting child health and development
- nursing sick children in partnership with families, educating children and their families
- helping families with a child with disability, complex needs or life-limiting illness
- treating children with acute or chronic health needs
- treating children with mental-health needs
- neonatal care (ill or premature newborn babies)
- paediatric (children's) emergency care.

Placements

Experiences will vary according to specific universities and Healthcare Trusts, but they will usually include a wide range of ages, from babies to teenagers. Settings can include:

- hospitals – in a range of wards including intensive care, high-dependency care and, in some areas, dedicated children's hospitals
- community – school nursing, health visiting, children's hospice and nurseries.

You can expect to have several placement experiences in community settings, reflecting the gradual shift in children's healthcare away from acute hospitals. You will be supervised and mentored mostly by experienced children's nurses.

Mental-health nursing

Mental-health nurses work with a range of ages, from children to adults, and with those with both physical and mental-health problems, ranging from anxiety to severe personality disorders. In this branch of nursing there is a focus on developing good communication skills, including therapeutic communication and assessment and intervention strategies.

You will learn about inter-agency and collaborative working, with social workers, psychologists, physiotherapists and occupational therapists and with third-sector and service-user organisations. Whilst retaining their independence as registered nurses and accountability for their practice, mental-health nurses frequently share responsibility for their clients with an extended multidisciplinary team. These teams often share a single client assessment – looking at health, mental, social and other needs – and plan and deliver care or services together. This requires high standards of communication and flexible working.

Person-centred care is also very important and courses will cover understanding the needs of users of mental-health services and looking at people as individuals, who experience mental-health problems in different ways.

As well as the general nursing modules outlined earlier in the chapter, courses may include:

- human behaviour, psychological approaches, abnormal psychology, personality and individual differences
- positive approaches to challenging behaviour
- communication strategies, including for the very vulnerable
- safeguarding patients, including safe administration of medication
- working to support individual rights and anti-discrimination, advocacy for clients and families
- assessment strategies and practices
- therapeutic interventions
- promoting positive mental and physical health messages and behaviours
- mental-health drugs
- working with adults of working age
- working with older adults, dementia care
- forensic nursing (working with offenders and those at risk of offending)
- acute mental problems
- ongoing mental-health problems
- drug and alcohol addiction
- eating disorders
- anxiety, depression, psychosis.

Placements

A range of opportunities should help you gain insight into, and experience of, the breadth of mental-health nursing provision in your local area. Experiences will vary but should include a wide range of ages, including children, teenagers and the elderly. You should gain experience of a range of dependences, from fully independent to full physical and mental dependence, and a range of behaviours, including challenging behaviour, addictions and perhaps working with offenders.

You will gain experience where clients are based: sometimes this will be in hospitals in acute or critical care, primary-care settings, such as GP surgeries or residential care, but it will most frequently be in the community or clients' homes.

Work may be with clients being cared for by the NHS, such as geriatric wards (dementia sufferers), acute psychiatric hospitals or in-patient units for children and adolescents. Experience can also be in local-authority community mental-health teams, such as crisis-intervention teams, children and adolescents teams, outreach services for those with long-term mental-health problems, drug and alcohol teams, learning-disability services and eating-disorder teams. It could also be in the prison service, or for private organisations or charities.

You can expect to be supervised and mentored by both experienced mental-health nurses and other relevant professionals.

Learning-disability nursing

Courses focus on learning to help people with learning disabilities participate in society and lead independent lives. This can include helping with daily-living activities, like dressing and shopping, to more complex issues, such as bringing up children. Learning disabilities can cause both mental and physical problems, from mild to severe, and learning-disability nurses often help clients deal with and manage a combination of physical, social and psychological or mental-health problems. The course may include multidisciplinary study alongside social-care courses. You will learn to work in partnership with service users and carers to make shared decisions and to work in inter-professional teams to make a single client assessment, considering health, mental, social and other needs, and then planning and delivering care or services together.

As well as the general nursing modules listed earlier in the chapter, courses may include:

- history of attitudes and values to people with learning disabilities
- identifying diverse and complex needs
- assessment, care plans and ongoing evaluation
- safeguarding clients, including safe administration of medication
- working to support individual rights and anti-discrimination
- supporting people with challenging behaviour
- forensic nursing (working with offenders and those at risk of offending).

Placements

You will gain insight into, and experience of, the range of clients receiving learning-disability nursing care in the local area. Experiences will normally include a wide range of ages, dependences and behaviours, including working with people who exhibit challenging behaviour.

You could work in a range of community settings, in family homes, residential and day services, schools, prisons, working for the NHS, a local authority or with private organisations or charities.

You can expect to be supervised and mentored by experienced learning-disability nurses, and service users (learning-disability clients) and carers may help with teaching and assessment, acting as 'experts through experience'.

Case study

Charlotte Hings is a third-year learning-disability nursing student at De Montfort University.

My current placement is for 10 weeks with an outreach team of community learning-disability nurses. These nurses support people with learning disabilities who are displaying challenging behaviours. The work involves observing clients in a variety of environments, such as college, their home or respite care to identify the 'triggers' that lead to challenging behaviours. For example someone with autism can become very anxious without a set routine, and unexpected requests or events can trigger off challenging behaviour. Once identified, a care plan with guidelines can be put in place to help that person actively manage the behaviours. Guidelines can be very detailed and are personal to each person. We also work with families and carers to put these guidelines into place.

The most challenging placement I have done so far has been working in a medium-secure hospital. I initially found it upsetting seeing someone being secluded and this made me quite emotional. Seclusion is where a person is restrained for their own and others' safety, and then taken into a seclusion room until their anxiety levels have decreased and they no longer pose a risk to themselves or others.

One of the most enjoyable aspects of being on placement has been learning to give a 'depot' injection. A depot injection is a form of a slow-release medication that can be given fortnightly to regulate a person's behaviours. This is one of the key clinical procedures learning-disability nurses learn to give and it is satisfying to know I am now competent to administer this.

I also enjoyed a 10-week placement at a respite care home as I was able to interact with many different patients with different types of learning disabilities. Respite care offers short-break residential care for patients away from their families or carers. They can return at various times of the year, so you can build up professional relationships with patients.

Midwifery

Courses have a focus on learning to provide individualised care and support to women and families to help them make choices about childbirth and caring for a baby. The course may begin with the study of normal pregnancy, labour and birth and lead on to more complicated maternity issues. You will learn to work in interdisciplinary teams. As well as the general nursing and midwifery course modules listed earlier in the chapter, courses may include:

- communication strategies, including where English is not spoken
- advocacy for mothers of all cultures/ethnicities and variations in midwifery practice
- antenatal and post-natal assessments
- health and parenting education
- normal pregnancy and childbirth
- complex pregnancy and complications in childbirth
- medical disorders encountered by childbearing women
- decision making in midwifery
- emergency-situation management
- pharmacology for midwifery
- continuity of care
- neonatal care (newborn and premature babies)
- newborn assessment
- promoting positive health messages to women and families (e.g. giving up smoking, sexual health).

Placements

Placements include hospital maternity wards, delivery suites, midwife-led birth centres, health centres, midwife-led community units, clients' homes and children's centres. Experience will be gained in both community and maternity hospital settings. You may have weekend, night and on-call duties. As your course develops, you may take increasing levels of responsibility, under supervision, for a number of normal and complex births as well as antenatal and post-natal assessments and associated care. You will normally be supervised and mentored by experienced midwives.

By the final placement there is quite a lot of responsibility. The NMC sets a requirement that students in their third year should have a caseload of women. Our students select three or four women that they look after all the way through, from booking to post-natal discharge. At all times they are accountable to a qualified midwife; they do not have sole responsibility. They attend antenatal appointments, possibly in partnership with a qualified midwife, are present for the birth wherever possible, and they can make visits to women and babies at home on their own with indirect supervision. On the delivery suite they are expected to manage labour and birth and make the plan of care, with a qualified midwife popping in and out and present for the birth. On antenatal wards and post-natal wards they are expected to manage a number of women and this might include delegating tasks to the maternity care assistant, under the watchful eye of a qualified midwife.

Heather Bower, Lead Midwife for Education
at Oxford Brookes University

Finding nursing and midwifery courses

Use the UCAS course search at www.ucas.com to locate pre-registration degree and pre-registration postgraduate diploma courses and the 'Apply' section of the website to make an application. For application to master's level courses, a small number of universities use UKPass, a service provided by UCAS, which also has a search facility. See www.ukpass.ac.uk.

For other courses you could use the postgraduate course search at www.prospects.ac.uk. The NHS course finder allows you to search for healthcare courses at all levels and includes full-time, part-time and in-service courses, see www.nhscareers.nhs.uk.

Access to nursing and midwifery courses

Access to Higher Education Diploma courses in nursing and/or midwifery are available at further-education colleges specifically for mature students (usually 19+) who want to improve their study skills, or return to study, to pursue a career in nursing or midwifery. The courses cover science, health studies, sociology, psychology, and study skills in English, maths and IT. Some courses offer work experience (or help you source your own experience) to support your application to university. Entry requirements may include GCSEs at C in maths and English, or literacy and numeracy tests may be used at interview to assess an applicant's ability to cope with the course. Pre-access courses are sometimes available if applicants are unsuccessful.

Applications should be made directly to further-education colleges. Many further-education colleges have good links with local nursing-degree courses and help and support are given with getting a place on a degree.

Bear in mind that there are fees for these courses and that they are not funded by NHS bursaries. However, you should speak to your local further-education college about fee concessions and other funding opportunities.

The Access course really helped to get me back into being in an educational environment. Being back in the classroom after 12 years was quite daunting but we were eased into the transition quite smoothly and the support from tutors was second to none.

The Access course prepared me well for my current midwifery degree. The units I studied were all relevant to midwifery and I especially found health studies fascinating and have used much of what I learnt in those lessons in my everyday clinical practice on placement. I know how to structure and reference an essay and have a really good grasp of anatomy, which helps, because in the first year we focus on it a lot. We also had tutorials on writing personal statements and I believe this was one of the main reasons I was offered an interview at my current university.

Donna McCarthy, first-year midwifery student
at the University of Bedfordshire

Apprenticeships

NHS Trusts sometimes offer apprenticeships in health, where you are based in a hospital and train as a healthcare assistant. It may then be possible to progress to a nursing degree, possibly through sponsorship from the NHS. Vacancies are occasionally advertised on www.jobs.nhs.uk.

3| Work experience

It is important to get relevant work experience before applying for a nursing or midwifery degree for several reasons. First, before starting a three-year vocational course, you need to be sure that this is the right career direction for you. You need to be sure that you want a job where the focus is on caring for people, have a realistic view of what nurses or midwives do and the settings in which they work. The best way to test this is to spend time in a care role, even if only on a short work placement or as a volunteer, spending time in a hospital or healthcare setting, talking to nurses and midwives about their jobs and how they feel about them, to gain a realistic insight into whether you would like this sort of work. You also need to test which branch of nursing would be right for you, by getting experience of working with clients typical to the branch in which you are interested. This is particularly important for mental-health nursing and learning-disability nursing.

Second, all pre-registration courses in nursing and midwifery will expect you to have gained some experience and skills related to your chosen profession before you apply, to demonstrate your motivation and commitment. You will be expected to discuss your work experience in your personal statement and at interview. Work experience can be full-time or part-time, paid or unpaid, and it can be fitted around other aspects of your life such as education and family commitments.

This chapter will help you identify the value of work experience and how you can apply this experience to making a successful application for a nursing or midwifery degree. It will also look at types of experience useful for each branch of nursing and midwifery and how to go about finding and applying for work experience.

Benefits of work experience

Some of the benefits of work experience are that you can:

- gain a realistic insight into particular job roles and work environments
- engage with current practitioners, with the chance to ask them about their jobs
- be introduced to the patient/client group(s) with whom you may want to work
- experience the highs and lows of working in healthcare and ask nurses and midwives what they like and dislike about their jobs

- confirm that you like an area of work before you commit yourself to a course; you may equally learn that a type of work isn't for you!
- open your eyes to other related jobs you hadn't previously considered
- be helped to decide whether you want to work in healthcare or social care (or a mixture of both)
- gain valuable experience for your CV or for an application to a course or job
- gain transferable skills, such as communication skills, teamworking, meeting deadlines
- network – making contacts for possible future work or making a good impression, so that you get a good reference or may be taken on again.

What counts as work experience?

Most nursing and midwifery courses will recommend as part of their entry requirements that you gain some relevant work experience before making an application and you will need to check carefully with each university about the nature of this requirement. Some may ask for general care experience, whilst others will ask for experience that shows you have transferable skills essential for nursing or midwifery, such as communication skills. Others may be more prescriptive and ask specifically for experience in healthcare, nursing or midwifery.

In the current economic climate you may find that you are competing for work experience (and even voluntary work) with many other people, including those who are keen to get experience as a way into employment or back into work. University admissions departments are aware of this and may be more flexible in the types of experience they will accept, especially if you are under 18, where finding relevant healthcare experience can be even more difficult. It is important to bear in mind that what counts as relevant experience can be much broader than you may think.

The comments from an admissions tutor and a first-year student that follow illustrate that what is most important is being proactive in getting experience and being able to show what you have gained from it.

We are looking for the whole picture – it's a lot more than just working at the local hospital – relevant experience can be much broader and can include observing and talking to qualified or student nurses and midwives, going to university open days and nursing and midwifery taster days, appropriate school work placements, going to study days and conferences and getting involved in groups and societies, such as NCT and La Leche League (breastfeeding support). It's how much they have gone out

there and put themselves forward and what they have gained from
these experiences.

Luisa Acosta, Senior Midwifery Lecturer and Admissions
Co-ordinator at the University of West London

I found it difficult to find work experience relevant to midwifery,
particularly because I was under 18. However, I managed to work-
shadow my uncle, who is an osteopath, once a week for three
months. I was worried that this experience would not be relevant
for getting on to a midwifery degree but was told by the university
I was applying to that it could be valid as long as I showed in my
personal statement how my experiences related to working as
a midwife. I was able to show I had an insight into a healthcare
role, the importance of respecting a patient's dignity and saw how
the osteopath reassured patients who were frightened about the
treatment they were about to receive.

Holly Janine Bexson Smith, first-year student
at De Montfort University

The following, from the University of York, is fairly typical of the sort of
experience universities state on their websites that they are looking for:

You may consider working in a nursing home, undertaking work-
shadowing at a local hospital or working for a voluntary organisa-
tion. The experience can be very varied but should demonstrate
your ability to work with others, communicate well and that you are
keen to learn more about the role you are entering into.

Source: www.york.ac.uk/healthsciences/nursing/faqs

In reality, as entry to courses is competitive, particularly for midwifery
and children's nursing, the more relevant the experience is, and the
more you can include the skills and insights you have learnt from it in
your personal statement (and at interview), the more you will have a
competitive edge. We will look at how to present your work experience
and transferable skills in Chapter 6.

How to find work experience

First of all, check whether your school or college allocates a specific
time when you are expected to go out on work experience (possibly a
one-week or two-week block) and whether you have to find your own
placement or are offered support with this. Your school or college may
have relationships with local hospitals and healthcare employers and

may be able either to find a placement for you or to advise you on how you should apply.

Hospital Trusts sometimes offer opportunities for 16-year-olds to spend time observing in certain areas of a hospital, but this can be limited and is unlikely to include maternity wards or children's wards. Work-experience schemes of this type increasingly ask students to make a personal application rather than schools applying on their behalf and may also require an interview. Look on Hospital Trust websites for information (you will find a listing of Hospital Trusts at www.nhs.uk/ServiceDirectories/Pages/AcuteTrustListing.aspx). Bear in mind that the experience you will gain may be limited to observing and it can be equally valuable to undertake (and easier to arrange) some voluntary experience in a care home or nursing home. This is often valued more highly by admissions tutors for applications to nursing and midwifery courses because you can gain hands-on experience of basic care skills.

If you cannot find any work-experience schemes advertised in your area, you may need to make speculative enquiries to relevant organisations, such as residential and care homes and charities to find possible opportunities. We will look at writing a suitable CV and covering letter for this purpose later in this chapter (see page 35). You could also look at websites that offer opportunities for work experience or voluntary work in the UK, such as www.vinspired.com, or abroad, such as World-wide Volunteering (www.wwv.org.uk), or seasonal work, such as www. seasonworkers.com.

Types of work experience

Volunteering

Many schools and colleges provide the opportunity for students to get involved in volunteering in healthcare and social care organisations, such as local care homes for the elderly or in local schools. Find out what is available if you are still in education – getting involved in such schemes will certainly give you experience of basic care skills; this is often what universities want and is an opportunity to test whether a care role is for you.

You could get in touch with relevant healthcare charities such as the Red Cross (www.redcross.org.uk), who offer care-in-the-home volunteering or Help the Hospices (www.helpthehospices.org.uk), where you can search for adult or children's hospices local to you, where you may be able to volunteer. Hospices are residential homes for people with life-limiting or terminal illness.

You can use the NHS Choices website to find NHS Trusts in your area and on these websites you should be able to find contact details for volunteering, either through the HR, voluntary-services or education-and-training departments. Hospitals may offer ward-visitor, 'meeter-greeter' or midwife 'buddy' type opportunities.

If you are 18 or over, you can volunteer as a community first responder for St John Ambulance (www.sja.org.uk), after first being trained in basic first-aid skills. There are also opportunities for under-18s to learn first-aid skills on cadet schemes. Be aware that this experience is directly related to being a paramedic and you should demonstrate on your personal statement that you understand the differences between a career as a nurse and that of an ambulance worker.

Helping out with a scout or guide group can be a valuable way of gaining people skills, and of working with children. You could also consider Community Service Volunteers (CSV), (www.csv.org.uk) who offer mentoring and befriending volunteer schemes, which include providing friendship to old people, supporting an at-risk family or supporting a person with a disability.

If you want to volunteer independently, many towns and cities in the UK have a volunteer centre that can put you in touch with relevant charities to which you could offer your time. See Volunteering England (www.volunteering.org.uk) for a list of volunteer centres and also Do-it (www.do-it.org.uk), which features volunteering opportunities through-out the UK.

There are many organisations, such as www.gapyear.com, that can arrange voluntary work for you in the UK or abroad, either as part of a gap year or as a summer job. These can be costly and you should look carefully at what is covered by the fee you pay, as it may not cover flights or travel insurance. Some organisations offer the chance to experience healthcare in developing countries and this can be very valu-able experience for a course application.

Paid employment

Paid employment in healthcare is an excellent way of gaining valuable experience but may be more difficult to find as well as being subject to age restrictions. As a preparation for nursing, working as a healthcare assistant can be very useful, and working as a maternity care assistant can be useful for midwifery. However, failing this, any hospital-based experience, such as working as a porter or administrative work, would be useful and allow you to speak to patients or get a feel for hospital working procedures. Use www.nhs.jobs.uk to find hospital-based vacancies. Care homes for the elderly often have vacancies for care assistants: look for vacancies in your local paper. A wide range of char-ities, such as Carewatch (www.carewatch.co.uk), employ care workers to support people in their own homes.

Any work where you can gain transferable people skills, teamwork or communication skills will also be valuable, for example, retail or catering.

You could look at seasonal vacation work, perhaps working on a local-authority play scheme or on a summer camp, such as Camp America, or sports camp, such as those run by PGL for young people.

Work experience in specific areas

Adult nursing

There are numerous opportunities for gaining experience working with adults who have additional needs – physical, social or emotional. In addition to formal work experience in hospitals or care institutions, considerable insight into the needs of frail or unwell adults can be gained from voluntary work. It is well worth approaching local nursing or residential homes, day centres and support groups (for example, for people who have had a stroke). NHS Trusts often offer voluntary work in a number of departments relating to care of adults, and you may be able to talk to patients, assist with meals and bed making and have the chance to shadow nurses taking blood pressure, temperature, completing fluid charts, etc. You could also consider charities that help specific groups, such as Age Concern and Victim Support.

The following comments from admissions tutors to adult nursing courses may give you an idea of the range of experience that can be relevant:

> Work experience needs to be care-related. We know it is difficult for younger students, straight from school, to access work experience in healthcare settings, but they can access domiciliary care (care in a person's home) or voluntary work in nursing homes and hospices. Experience in retail, waitressing or any activities such as the Duke of Edinburgh Scheme or being a peer mentor can show communication skills, leadership and organisation skills and are all valid if transferable skills are identified and shown how they are valuable to adult nursing. Applicants can build up quite a strong personal statement even if they haven't had a lot of direct care experience.
>
> Sally Morey, admissions tutor for adult nursing
> at Oxford Brookes University

> We like to see that applicants have done some type of experience, preferably in a nursing care setting.
>
> Fiona Bazoglu, admissions officer for nursing
> at the University of Edinburgh

Children's nursing

Many applicants for children's nursing have experience of working with healthy children, for example, babysitting; work experience in a nursery; helping in a local primary school; summer play schemes; volunteering at scouts and guides; work in a youth club; or a summer job with an organisation that offers activity holidays for children, such as PGL or Camp America. This is certainly helpful, but children's nurses are involved in caring for sick children and working with their families. Where possible, it is useful to gain experience with children who do not enjoy normal health. Work experience in hospital children's wards is not usually possible but some hospitals offer chances to volunteer, for example, organising activities for children waiting for A&E. Volunteering for a local charity that supports children with special needs or a disability is very useful; these children may have associated health issues.

Mental-health nursing and learning-disability nursing

An insight into the needs of people with learning disabilities or mental-health issues can be gained most easily from voluntary work. Many nursing homes offer professional nursing care for people with dementia and a wide range of other mental-health needs. Similarly, residential settings, sometimes managed by charities or local authorities, offer extended care for people with learning disabilities. Many such nursing and residential settings greatly appreciate volunteers, who in turn gain insight into the reality of client care and can see nurses in action. Time permitting, a regular weekly commitment for six months or more could give you the potential to build an understanding of the duties and roles undertaken in these branches of nursing. You could also consider voluntary work for a mental-health charity, such as Mind (www.mind.org.uk) or a learning-disability charity, such as Mencap (www.mencap.org.uk).

Midwifery

University admissions departments are aware that finding work experience in midwifery is difficult, especially for those under 18. Some will make allowances for this and will not insist on midwifery experience but suggest you gain general healthcare experience or at least work with adults in a way that you can demonstrate has helped you develop skills useful for midwifery.

> *We do look for work experience, but not necessarily in midwifery. Work experience in a healthcare setting would be ideal, even if this is only voluntary work, to get a taste of working in a multi-professional healthcare team, or at least seeing one in action. However, work experience or voluntary work in a GP's surgery, children's centre, care home, learning-disabilities setting or*

with the public are all valid. Anything they have done which demonstrates they have improved their communication skills is good. What we'd like to know is that they can see the relevance of the work experience – not just telling us they have done it, but drawing links as to how it might help them in a future midwifery role. We would also expect them to have talked to a midwife, to see what it is like on the inside.

Heather Bower, Lead Midwife for Education
at Oxford Brookes University

Most courses will expect you to have at least talked to a midwife and found out about what they actually do day to day. Practising midwives are sometimes inundated with requests for work-shadowing or experience from aspiring midwifery students, so you must bear in mind that they may not be able or willing to help. You can use the independent midwives website, www.independentmidwives.org.uk to locate independent midwives in your area, who may be more willing to answer your questions. However, you will probably find that either a family member or friend will know a midwife – you may be able to shadow them at work or, if this is not possible due to patient confidentiality, ask them questions away from the workplace about what their job entails.

Work experience is not usually possible in hospital maternity departments due to the nature of the work, but any hospital-based work where you have a chance to talk to and support adult female patients will be useful. Also consider charities relating to midwifery, such as the National Childbirth Trust (NCT) and Bliss (www.bliss.org.uk) that support families with sick or premature babies. Use www.nct.org.uk to find details of your local NCT branch to offer help at antenatal classes or post-natal breastfeeding-support group.

If you really can't find any specific maternity-related work experience, think about the skills midwives need: being able to communicate in stressful circumstances; teamwork skills; tolerance; trustworthiness; advocacy skills; and knowledge of public-health issues – find work experience to show that you have developed these skills.

Although there are increasing numbers of students applying to midwifery directly from school or college and universities are welcoming this, you need to bear in mind that many applicants to midwifery courses are mature students, who may be changing career and already have a lot of relevant work and life experience. If you are a younger applicant, you are up against this competition and really need to show your commitment to midwifery by being proactive to find some relevant experience.

How to apply for work experience

If an employer, such as an NHS Trust, advertises on their website that they offer work experience, you will have to follow their guidelines carefully on how to apply. They may ask you to complete an application form or to contact them by email with some details about yourself and a statement about why you want to apply for a particular type of work experience.

Putting together a CV

If you are contacting an employer speculatively to enquire whether they offer work experience or voluntary work, you should send a CV and covering letter. It's never too early to start to put together a CV, useful for applying for work experience or part-time work. This is a summary of relevant details about your qualifications, work experience, interests and achievements to date and can be either one or two pages long, depending on how much work experience you have. If you are a mature student having had a lot of jobs, you will probably need to use two pages.

You should include the following on a CV:

- name, address and contact details
- date of birth
- education and qualifications
- interests/positions of responsibility/achievements
- skills
- referees.

Education and qualifications

Start with your current school/college and what you are studying at the moment and the qualifications for which you intend to sit. Then list any previous secondary schools and the qualifications you gained with grades and dates. Use bullet points to highlight any subjects or projects particularly relevant to nursing or midwifery.

Work experience

Start with the most recent experience. Don't worry if you've only had a Saturday job at the local shop or done a paper round or babysitting. Put it all down and try to draw out any specific skills you have gained from it, such as communication skills, working in a team, working with the public and so on, relevant to the work experience you are seeking.

Interests/positions of responsibility/achievements

What do you like to do in your spare time? Try to show that you are a well-rounded person who takes part in a range of activities both in and out of school and that some of your interests relate to nursing or midwifery, such as befriending or doing odd jobs for an elderly neighbour. Don't forget to detail any positions of responsibility or where you have had to lead others, such as being captain of a sports team, a prefect or school-council member.

Skills

List any additional skills relevant to nursing or midwifery, such as first aid, computer skills and possessing a driving licence.

Referees

It is acceptable to put 'References available on request' at the bottom of your CV and then on a separate sheet keep names, addresses and contact details of two people who would be happy to write a reference (a statement about the sort of person you are) for you if needed. The first referee usually needs to be an academic referee, such as a tutor/teacher or head teacher; and the second, an employer you have worked for, or someone who knows you well personally, who is not a relative.

Below is an example of how you can present your CV.

A sample CV

Sophie Tate
134 Hillhouse Avenue
Portsmouth PO1 2TQ
01234 567890
07787 112 977
tates@btinternet.com
d.o.b. 10 June 1996

Education & qualifications
Linfield High School, Portsmouth
2007–present

A levels
Biology, Sociology, English

GCSEs
English literature (A), English language (A), Mathematics (B), History (A), Geography (C), Chemistry (B), Biology (B), French (A), ICT (D)

Positions of responsibility/achievements
- Captain of B netball team.
- Year representative for school council, suggesting ideas to improve school life.

- Completed Duke of Edinburgh Bronze Award, including expedition and community involvement – washed cars for elderly neighbours to raise money for charity for bereaved children. Duke of Edinburgh Silver Award in progress.
- Taught primary-school children to play netball for sports-leadership award.

Employment
2011 (Saturdays) to present
Sales assistant – Sava Supermarket

- Improving my communication skills, helping customers use self-service tills.
- Working in chilled foods team, to keep shelves stocked.

Babysitting (ongoing)

- Looking after a wide age range from babies up to a six-year-old.

Work experience
3–7 May 2010
Seaview Care Home, Portsmouth

- Talking to residents and playing cards/board games.
- Helping serve meals.

Skills

- Computing – competent in MS Word and Excel.
- St John Ambulance cadet scheme – learning first aid.

Interests
Netball, swimming, playing drums in a band.
References available on request.

Tips for your CV

- There is no standard CV and you can change the order and titles of section headings according to what you think is the most important information, i.e. the information that you want the employer to see first.
- Always highlight your good points on a CV – don't be negative and only include things you would be happy to talk about at interview.
- If something, such as illness, prevented you from reaching your potential in your exams, point this out in the covering letter (see below).

The covering letter

CVs should always be accompanied by a covering letter. The letter is important because it is usually the first thing an employer reads so you need to make sure you explain why you are contacting them and why they should read your CV.

Here are some tips.

- You can send it by post or email as long as you have the correct contact details.
- The letter should be on the same type of A4 plain paper as your CV if you are sending by post and should be one page/side of A4 only.
- Try to find out the name of the person to whom you should send or email your letter and CV. It is far more likely to be read. If you start the letter 'Dear Mr Brown', remember that you should finish it 'Yours sincerely'.
- The first paragraph should tell the reader why you are contacting them.
- The second paragraph should give them some information to make them interested in you, e.g. highlighting your interest in nursing along with some relevant experience.

A sample covering letter is shown below.

Dear Mrs Smith,

I am writing to enquire whether you may be in a position to offer any work experience at Portsmouth Nursing Home during the Easter holidays. I am currently studying A levels at Linfield High School and interested in applying for degrees in adult nursing next September.

I am keen to gain practical experience of working with adults, particularly those with medical needs, developing basic care skills and improving my communication skills. I have already spent a week at a care home talking to residents and playing games with them, so have some experience of talking to people of this age group. I know that you employ qualified adult nurses and I would like if possible to observe them at work and help with basic nursing duties.

I am available from 1 to 15 April. I look forward to hearing from you and please do not hesitate to contact me if you would like me to provide references.

Yours sincerely,

Sophie Tate

What to look for during work experience

Work experience can provide you with invaluable opportunities to develop your knowledge and understanding of nursing and midwifery as a career. It is therefore vital that you pay close attention to what is going on around you so that you can get the most from the experience. It is a good idea to carry a notebook and pen so that you can jot down answers to questions you have asked as well as any thoughts or observations related to your experiences. In addition, it is worth trying to keep a diary of what you have observed as this will be really useful when it comes to writing a personal statement for your UCAS application and for attending interviews.

Show an interest in all that is going on around you and offer to help with routine tasks, so that you give the employer something in return for the useful insight you get into the job.

During your placements, pay attention to the following aspects of nursing, midwifery or healthcare practice.

Skills that nurses/midwives need

Nurses and midwives need a wide range of skills to do their job effectively; it is therefore a good idea to keep a note of the range of personal qualities nurses or midwives demonstrate on a day-to-day basis as well as the variety of tasks they carry out. This will help provide you with a list of the sort of skills you will need to develop and can talk about in interviews.

Interactions with patients

A vital part of a nurse/midwife's role is to interact with patients, to find out how they are feeling, what their needs are and to answer questions and reassure them. Take time to observe how healthcare workers communicate with patients, particularly those who are anxious about being treated.

The variety of treatments available to patients

Make sure that you know what you are observing during your placement. Ask for the technical names of the procedures you see and for information on the equipment used. Ask about the advantages and disadvantages of different types of treatment.

The roles of different team members

In any setting, there will be a wide range of individuals involved who are vital to the overall functioning of the team. For example, in addition to the nurses there will also be healthcare assistants, doctors, care workers and administrators. Make sure that you take time to talk to as many members of the team as possible and ask them about the role they play.

Working as a nurse or midwife

Ask the nurse/midwife about their job. Find out about the hours, the way in which they are paid, the demands of the job and the career options. Find out what they like and dislike about the job.

Ultimately, being observant and asking questions will help you further your understanding of what is required to be a nurse/midwife. At the end of each of your placements, you should ask yourself whether this is still a career path that you wish to pursue. If there are any aspects of the work that you dislike, you should be honest with yourself and consider whether these would put you off becoming a nurse/midwife.

Work-shadowing

If it is difficult to find experience in a specific branch of nursing or midwifery, see whether you can work-shadow someone instead. Work-shadowing involves spending time observing someone in an occupation that interests you, without a practical involvement.

Use work-shadowing as an opportunity to ask questions about the job that you are observing. Before meeting the person that you will be shadowing, make a list of questions to ask them as this will make your meeting far more constructive. The questions could include the following.

- Why did you decide to become a nurse or midwife?
- What nursing/midwifery jobs have you had so far?
- What do you like/dislike about your current job?
- What do you find challenging about your current job?
- What hours do you work?
- What is your working environment like?
- Who do you work with?
- In your opinion, what are the skills and qualities that you need to be an effective nurse/midwife?

With some relevant experience and knowledge under your belt you will be in a better position to both choose and apply for nursing and midwifery courses – the topic of the next chapter.

4 | Choosing your course

In this chapter we will look at the factors you need to take into account when choosing a nursing or midwifery course. The chapter will cover the entry requirements for different courses and how to choose a university, taking into account aspects such as location, size and cost. We will also consider the skills needed for each branch of nursing to further help you make the right decision as to which branch will be best for you.

You can apply for up to five courses on your UCAS application. The basic factors to consider when choosing degree courses are:

- your academic ability (what grades are you likely to get?)
- where you want to study
- what exactly you want to study (i.e. which branch of nursing).

Entry requirements

From September 2013, entry to nursing will be by degree only, so you must check that you will have the entry requirements necessary for degree-level study. Entry to midwifery is through the degree route only and is very competitive. The NMC provides guidance to universities on the standards and competencies students must attain by the end of their course but it is up to individual universities to set their own entry requirements, which can vary widely.

Minimum entry requirements

To study a course leading to registration as a nurse or a midwife, you will need the following entry requirements:

- five GCSEs at grade C or above to include English, maths and possibly a science subject.

In addition to:

- A levels or equivalent qualifications. The grades required by each university will vary widely. There may also be subject requirements, such as a science (see later in this chapter).

A wide range of equivalent qualifications are also accepted, including:

- SQA Highers and Advanced Highers
- Access to Higher Education Diploma
- BTEC National Certificate or Diploma in health and social care or applied science
- 14–19 Advanced Diploma
- International Baccalaureate or European Baccalaureate Diploma.

If you are studying a 14–19 Diploma or a BTEC National Certificate/ Diploma, you should check whether it is accepted on its own or whether it needs to be combined with additional qualifications such as a science A level. If you are at all unsure, phone or email university admissions departments to make sure that your A level choices or equivalents meet their entry requirements.

To study a postgraduate diploma leading to registration as a nurse or midwife, you will need a 2.ii degree or above in a subject relevant to nursing, such as biological sciences, social sciences, psychology, behavioural sciences or health studies. Check with individual universities to see whether your degree will be acceptable.

Typical offers

Universities will state their entry requirements in terms of the grades you will be expected to achieve to be successful in securing a place; in other words, the grades a university will typically require if they make you an offer. In setting their entry requirements for each course, universities often publish their grade and subject requirements at least a year ahead of the course's start date, in prospectuses for example. These requirements can change, so you should check individual university websites for any changes before you complete your UCAS application.

Universities may state their typical offers as grades or UCAS points. If you are unclear about UCAS points, see the UCAS Tariff on the UCAS website (www.ucas.com/students/ucas_tariff) for an explanation and to calculate how many points you could achieve. If you have any specific queries, it is always worth checking these out directly with university admissions tutors, for example, if you have made a previous application and are reapplying to the same university.

Universities often state typical offers but might adjust these in individual cases, for example, for a mature student with a lot of relevant work experience, so it is always worth contacting the admissions department to discuss individual circumstances if you're at all unsure.

There can be considerable variation in grade requirements between nursing and midwifery courses due to the popularity of each university and the numbers of applications for each course. You must check the typical entry requirements at each individual university for the qualifications you are taking. The following will give you an idea of the wide range of university entry requirements for nursing and midwifery pre-registration degree courses:

Nursing

- A level: from 260 points (BCC equivalent) to ABB
- International Baccalaureate: from 24 to 34 points
- BTEC National Diploma in health and social care or applied science: from MMM to DDM
- Scottish Higher/Advanced Highers: from BBB Advanced Highers or AABBB Highers to BBBB Highers
- Access to Higher Education Diploma: from 15 level 3 units at merit to 30 level 3 units at distinction in addition to 15 level 3 units at merit.

Midwifery

- A level: from 260 points (BCC equivalent) to AAB
- BTEC National Diploma in health and social care or science: from MMM to DDD
- International Baccalaureate: from 24 to 34 points
- Scottish Higher/Advanced Highers: from BBB Advanced Highers or AABBB Highers to BBBB Highers
- Access to Higher Education Diploma: from 15 level 3 units at merit to 30 level 3 units at distinction in addition to 15 level 3 units at merit.

Some universities will set higher grade requirements for children's nursing and midwifery due to the popularity of these courses. If you don't think you are adequately prepared for studying a degree course, you can either plan to upgrade your qualifications, by taking an Access or Health Foundation course (see Chapter 2 for more details about these courses), or consider employment as a healthcare assistant or midwifery care assistant.

Predicted grades

As you research universities, keep in mind your current grade level and ask your teachers/tutor for the grades they predict you should be able to achieve at A2 or equivalent qualifications and balance these against your own realistic ambitions. This will become easier when you have sat your AS levels or equivalent and have actual grades to base predictions on what you can realistically achieve at A2 or the completion of your course. You can then explore the typical entry grades for universities, using the UCAS course search at www.ucas.com or university websites or prospectuses and make a range of course choices that sit within the grades you can realistically achieve.

> **TIP**
>
> The most important thing is to be honest with yourself, however much you like the look of a university and course. If the typical grades or UCAS points requirement are higher than you are predicted to achieve, it may be a wasted choice on your application. You should aim to have a range of choices including one or two universities that you like where the grades are lower than you are predicted as a fall-back plan.

Subject requirements

To apply for a nursing or midwifery degree you will also need to have a certain level of ability in maths, English and science, in order to be able to cope with the demands of the course and because the NMC requires potential nurses and midwives to have competence in numeracy and literacy in order to practise.

Maths (numeracy)

For all nurses and midwives, accuracy in dispensing medicines and in calculating or checking dosages is essential. A misplaced decimal point could mean that a patient gets 10 times too much or 10 times too little medication – either could have very serious consequences. The issue is more than having an exam pass – it is about being comfortable with handling numbers.

The NMC states that the requirements for both nurses and midwives are that they must be competent at volume, weight and length using addition, subtraction, division and multiplication, use of decimals, fractions and percentages and use of a calculator. All approved nursing and midwifery courses must ensure that students can reach this requirement by the end of the course. They may set an entry requirement of a minimum grade C (in some cases grade B) in GCSE maths. Some universities will accept alternative number-related qualifications; you need to check with each individual university.

Universities may choose to check applicants' number skills by setting a numeracy test at the selection day and in some cases you need to pass this to go on to the interview stage. You will find more details about numeracy tests in Chapter 7.

English (literacy)

Good spoken and written communication skills are essential in nursing and midwifery. The NMC gives guidance to universities on the level of literacy skills required to practise as a nurse or midwife and universities will set entry requirements to ensure that applicants can reach that level. You will probably need GCSE English language grade C (some ask for grade B) although a number of alternative English-language qualifications are considered by some universities – check on an individual basis.

Universities may include a literacy test as part of the selection process. There are more details in Chapter 7.

If English is not your first language or your education was not in English, you will normally have to meet the requirement recommended by the NMC of a score of 7 in the IELTS (International English Language Testing System) or equivalent. This is not always clearly stated on university websites or prospectuses and is not to be confused with the general university-wide requirements for international students, which can be lower at 5.5 to 6.5. If you are in doubt, you should contact individual universities.

Science

All nursing and midwifery courses involve studying life sciences, anatomy and physiology, so universities will usually have science entry requirements. They may require science GCSE at C or require (or prefer) that you have a science A level (biology or human biology is usually preferred). If you have studied a BTEC National Diploma or 14–19 Diploma, there may also be a requirement to have studied a science at A level (usually biology or human biology). If you have studied an Access course, you may need credits at certain levels in biology, human biology, chemistry or science. You should check individual universities for their specific entry requirements.

Accreditation of prior (experiential) learning

You may be able to be accredited for previous relevant study (APL) or experience (APEL) in place of some of the university entrance requirements. Also, in theory, up to one third of a three-year programme can be accredited in this way, to shorten the length of a course, but it is at the discretion of each university. In practice, for pre-registration courses, universities may not be keen to allow this and may prefer all applicants to meet set academic standards and start the course at the beginning. You must bear in mind that APEL requires a great deal of time and work to put together a portfolio and that this must prove that you are exempt from practice because your work experience matches what nursing or midwifery students would encounter on placement. APL or APEL is more likely to be accepted by universities for post-registration courses.

Choosing a course or university

The best way to choose a course or university is to look at all the available information, from university prospectuses and websites, and to visit the universities to help decide which are right for you. The most important thing to keep in mind is that different places suit different people and that although many people can help you make a choice the end decision should be yours. Other information you may find useful for comparing and choosing courses and universities includes:

- UCAS course search at www.ucas.com.
- Key Information Sets – information relating to student satisfaction with courses and the quality of teaching, employment rates, costs of courses and accommodation, currently found on http://unistats. direct.gov.uk and which often appears next to each individual university's course details on university websites.
- The Complete University Guide, www.thecompleteuniversityguide. co.uk, includes university profiles with information on student facilities, academic strengths, accommodation costs and bursaries and scholarships.
- The Guardian University Guide, www.guardian.co.uk/education/ universityguide, has league tables for best universities for certain subjects according to such factors as student satisfaction.

Remember to use league tables as a rough guide and with care, and have an understanding of how they are compiled and the factors which have been taken into account.

You may also wish to consider the following factors when making your decision about where to study.

Finances

The cost of living is not the same across the UK; it is considerably higher in the south, particularly in London, and accommodation costs can vary widely. The NHS bursary is higher for students studying in London but you should remember that everything will be more expensive, even a cup of coffee.

Close to home?

Whilst there can be advantages to living at home, you might prefer the challenge of looking after yourself and the opportunity to be completely independent. Consider the costs of travel from university to home at the end of each term and if you want to pop back for weekends to visit friends and family.

Accommodation

Do you want to live in halls of residence with other students or in private housing? You may wish to check whether the university guarantees a room in halls of residence to all first-year students and what the cost would be. Bear in mind that you will probably have to fend for yourself at some stage, so check on the availability of student housing, the cost and the distance from the university.

Leisure and entertainment

If you have specific interests, such as sport or theatre, you may want to look for specific facilities or university societies.

Site and size

Check carefully the location of the university campus for the course you want to do. Some universities have several sites, some being a distance from the main site. Do you want to be in a city with direct access to all facilities and feel that you are part of a city community? Would you prefer to be on an out-of-town campus site, perhaps with easier access to the countryside? Campus sites are often like mini student towns, with all you need on one site. Many universities overcome the problems of urban versus rural and small versus large by locating their campuses on the edge of a major town. If a university is multi-site, how easy is it to travel between sites if you need to?

Facilities

Does the university have a good simulation suite, where you can practise clinical skills? Does it have good library resources and IT facilities?

University open days

Visit any universities you are considering applying to and use this opportunity to ask questions of staff and students. Don't just find out about the courses: also ask about the clinical placements, the accommodation and the social life. You will be spending three years on your higher-education course, so make sure that it suits you. Try to imagine what it would be like to study there. Can you see yourself living and working there? Current students and staff are often available to answer questions; talks and taster sessions may be on offer.

Look at individual university websites for information on open days. You will need to register and it is often first come, first served, for departmental tours and taster sessions.

After each visit to an open day it is a good idea to make notes of your impressions and what differences you spotted. These notes will be very useful if you are called for interview when you may be asked about your visit.

Choosing your branch of nursing

You will need to consider:

- your reasons or motivations for wanting to go into nursing or midwifery.
- your own personality: how do you 'get on' with different age groups/ different people's needs?
- experience: what have you learnt from your shadowing/work/ voluntary/employed experience? Try to gain experience in more than one setting if you are not certain.

You may find hospital open days useful to see different areas of nursing in action. Most large NHS Hospital Trusts offer open days where departmental staff are available to demonstrate and explain their roles. Check your local NHS Hospital Trust website.

The areas of nursing that you can choose are:

- adult nursing
- children's nursing
- mental-health nursing
- learning-disability nursing.

We will go on to look at the skills needed for each branch of nursing and for midwifery. Some of these are generic skills needed by all nurses or midwives but there are also specific skills needed relating to the client group with which you would be working. You may find it useful to consider these skills in conjunction with information on course content as detailed in Chapter 2 and the careers to which you can progress from each branch of nursing as detailed in Chapter 11.

What skills will I need?

To be a nurse you need to be:

- a good communicator who can listen and explain things clearly
- well organised
- observant and attentive to detail
- interested in caring for people and able to show empathy
- calm
- a good teamworker
- comfortable about dealing with personal care and bodily fluids (e.g. blood, urine)
- an effective problem-solver who can evaluate situations and see a way forward
- resilient: some days will be challenging as well as rewarding
- able to work independently, be responsible but recognising your boundaries and limits

- professional with personal integrity
- confident with writing and IT to complete records and care plans
- able to use theory and research findings to inform your work (evidence-based practice)
- interested in promoting best practice and improvements to practice
- prepared to carry on studying after qualifying to keep yourself up to date.

The following are more specific skills and qualities, particularly important for each branch of nursing.

Adult nursing

Skills that adult nurses need include:

- excellent and sensitive verbal and non-verbal communication skills, confidence to talk to a variety of ages and sometimes in difficult circumstances
- the ability to consider social and psychological needs as well as health needs
- a genuine desire to be involved in personal care, including safeguarding vulnerable adults and the elderly and respecting dignity
- being able to work in partnership and make shared decisions with other healthcare professionals, families and carers
- the ability to engage sensitively with clients of all backgrounds, cultures and beliefs, be non-judgemental, respect individual differences and support social inclusion
- willingness to advocate for and promote the rights of patients
- being able to promote public health, be a role model and give advice and educate
- being able to use diagnostic skills and make assessments and decisions
- good observation skills, to be alert to even minor changes in patient condition
- physical and emotional stamina
- being prepared to take the lead in coordinating and delegating care.

Children's nursing

Skills that children's nurses need include:

- excellent and sensitive verbal and non-verbal communication skills
- being able to act as an advocate for children and negotiating with others on a child's behalf, as children cannot so easily articulate what they feel, involving children in decision making
- the ability to talk to a range of adults, to work in partnership with parents and carers, respond to distressed parents/carers in emotionally challenging situations and explain treatment clearly to enable parents and carers to consent to treatment

- being able to work in partnership and make shared decisions with other healthcare professionals, families and carers
- understanding child development, communicate appropriately with children according to their stage of development, use play and distraction techniques
- good observation skills, to be alert to even minor changes in patient condition, awareness of vulnerability of infants and young children to rapid physiological deterioration
- being able to promote healthy living and prevention of illness and injury, advising and educating parents
- having a responsible approach to safeguarding children
- consistency and reliability.

Mental-health nursing

Skills that mental-health nurses need include:

- excellent and sensitive verbal and non-verbal communication skills, good listening skills
- patience
- the ability to build relationships to gain people's trust to help them disclose and discuss experiences to aid recovery
- being prepared to work in multidisciplinary teams
- the ability to engage sensitively with clients of all backgrounds, cultures and beliefs
- the potential to cope with difficult or distressing situations, intervention and harm reduction, crisis resolution
- being prepared to work with people at risk of suicide and self-harm, responding to distressed patients
- an interest in promoting health and well-being, self-care, giving advice on drugs and treatments and side effects
- being positive and patient-recovery focused
- a genuine desire to be involved in personal care, including safeguarding vulnerable adults, respecting individual choices
- an awareness of own mental health and how your own values and beliefs affect how you work with others
- being happy to work both one-to-one with clients and run group sessions.

Learning-disability nursing

Skills that learning-disability nurses need include:

- excellent and sensitive verbal and non-verbal communication skills with a range of ages and social groups, good listening skills
- patience; as the rewards from interventions and care are often delayed
- being prepared to promote rights, choices and independence of those with disabilities, support clients to be independent

- the ability to consider social and psychological needs as well as health needs
- being able to build relationships with patients and gain their trust
- a genuine interest in all people whatever their disability
- a willingness to represent needs of people with learning disabilities, challenge discrimination and negative stereotypes
- emotional resilience
- being prepared to work in multidisciplinary teams
- the ability to engage sensitively with clients of all backgrounds, cultures and beliefs
- the potential to learn how to respond to distressed clients or those with challenging behaviour
- confidence in talking with people who cannot communicate or respond easily, flexibility to adapt means of communication or adapt information
- the potential to cope with difficult or distressing ethical situations
- being able to lead and coordinate individual patient care plans
- being able to plan and run group activities (in supported living settings).

Midwifery

Skills that midwives need include:

- excellent and sensitive verbal and non-verbal communication skills appropriate to different women, including those who do not speak English or have learning or sensory disabilities, good listening skills
- the ability to explain choices, benefits and risks of different birth options, give information and advice
- the ability to be non-judgemental and respect rights and choices of all women and their families irrespective of class, ethnicity, age, sexuality or beliefs
- an interest in pregnancy and birth, from a scientific, psychological and social perspective
- being confident and mature, someone who will make women feel positive and in control, ability to be directive when needed
- empathy, sensitivity and a warm caring personality
- the ability to work well independently and as a part of a multidisciplinary team
- being alert and a quick thinker, flexible to complications, able to remain calm and objective and able to react quickly in an emergency and be prepared to undertake emergency procedures
- physical and emotional stamina
- counselling skills – in difficult circumstances: miscarriage, termination, stillbirth, neonatal abnormality, neonatal death
- practical skills – able to combine practical and emotional support
- accuracy – to interpret screening tests, drug calculations.

Questions to consider when choosing a branch of nursing

Can I change between different areas of nursing?

In most cases this is not possible as pre-registration courses are very structured: it would depend on how far you were into a course and the availability of spaces on other branches. It is better to be absolutely sure of the branch of nursing you want to do before you apply. You could also consider a dual-registration course. It may be possible after you have qualified to choose a post-registration course to move towards another area of nursing but this will be dependent on the availability of post-registration courses in your area and funding from your employer, as NHS bursaries are not available for post-registration courses.

I really enjoy working with young children. Is midwifery or children's nursing more relevant?

A midwife's primary role is to support women through pregnancy, labour and childbirth and to help new mothers to look after their children – there is little direct childcare involved.

Children's nurses work with children who are ill, very ill or disabled by their health, who often behave very differently from healthy children.

If you want to work with healthy, well children, you could consider being an Early Years or primary teacher, a nursery nurse, nanny or play worker. Use work experience to find out the differences between working with well children and those that are ill.

What is best: a three-year or four-year course?

The majority of UK universities offer both nursing and midwifery as three-year courses, with some opportunities for a four-year course if you need more time and flexibility to complete your course, want to include postgraduate study, want dual registration or need extra foundation study before you start your degree. As what you need to learn to register and practise as a nurse or midwife will be roughly the same on each course, course length is a personal choice and it depends what is right for you and which courses you prefer. You should note that in Scotland it takes four years to complete an honours degree.

I think I might want to teach nursing/midwifery in the future or pursue a research career. Does my choice of course matter?

Nurses and midwives are employed as lecturers in universities (to teach and as researchers). University lecturers normally have a higher degree at master's or doctoral level. All nursing and midwifery courses could lead to teaching; it is likely that you will need at least several years of experience working in your field before full-time teaching becomes possible. Some pre-registration courses have more of an emphasis on learning research methods and skills or you may wish to consider a course that leads directly to a master's-level qualification.

5 | The UCAS application

Full-time pre-registration nursing degrees are offered at around 56 universities and midwifery degrees at around 42 universities throughout the UK. Applications to courses are made through UCAS. Applications to the pre-registration postgraduate diploma courses in nursing and midwifery are also made through UCAS. Visit www.ucas.com at least a year before applying and start to become familiar with the application process and deadlines.

If you are applying for a master's-level course, some universities use UKPass, a service provided by UCAS, or ask you to apply directly to the university.

Applications for all part-time courses should be made directly to the university and, for nursing courses with January starts, you may have to apply directly to the university as well as through UCAS. Check individual university admissions details carefully.

UCAS Apply

Applications are made through the UCAS Apply system, an online application process. You register online at www.ucas.com either through your school or college, or as a private individual. You need to provide some basic personal details to register and then you are given a username and create your own password.

If you apply to more than one course, university or college, the cost is currently £23. If you apply to only one course at one university or college, it is £12. Costs may go up each year, so check with www.ucas.com.

The application has a number of sections that need to be filled in and you can save each section as you go, logging in again when you want to add more details or amend details.

- **Personal details.** The basic details you provided at registration are automatically transferred into this section and you need to add a few extras, such as nationality and how the course is going to be funded. In nearly all cases you need to indicate that the course will be funded by an NHS bursary.
- **Choices.** You can choose up to five courses at one or more universities. It is not a good idea to apply for more than one nursing or midwifery course at a single university as this will not signal your

commitment to a branch of nursing and will indicate that you have not taken the time to research and decide which branch is best for you. It will also be very difficult to write a good personal statement if you are still undecided. See Chapter 6 for further guidance on this. If you apply to fewer than five choices, you can add further choices up to 30 June. Pay particular attention to the course codes and university codes, and ensure that all of the required information, such as where you intend to live and to which campus you are applying, is included.

- **Education.** Provide details of schools and colleges where you have studied, your examination results and any examinations to be sat. Check that you have included all of the courses you are currently studying.
- **Employment.** Include part-time work, Saturday jobs, even if you don't think these are relevant to the course you want to do. Universities like to see that you have some work experience, and remember that all jobs are useful for transferable skills. If you have had gaps in your education because you were in employment, the job details need to be here.
- **Personal statement.** This is one of the most important parts of the application. See Chapter 6 for guidance on how to complete this.
- **Reference.** Once you have completed all of these sections, you will need to click on the appropriate section to send the form to your referee, so that they can add their comments about your suitability for your chosen courses. Your referee is normally someone at your school or college, such as a personal tutor or head of sixth form. For applicants who are not at school, this might be an employer or someone who is not a relative who knows you well. The referee then sends the application on to UCAS and after that, you can keep track of how your application is progressing and the responses from the universities you have chosen on the UCAS online Track facility.

> You may find it useful to have further information, tips and advice about how best to complete your application. *How to Complete Your UCAS Application 2014 Entry* (Trotman) provides detailed information.

When to submit the UCAS application

The closing date for sending an application to UCAS for nursing and midwifery courses is 15 January. However, you must remember that this is the deadline by which the form must arrive at UCAS. Your school or college will have an earlier deadline so that they have time to write and input your reference onto the application. You must check with your school or college the date by which you need to have completed all the sections of your form and have sent it to your referee.

Applications received after the deadline and up until 30 June will be considered by universities or colleges only if they still have vacancies for the course you have selected. As nursing and midwifery courses are very popular, for many universities it is unlikely that late applications will be considered.

TIP

Although you can submit your application at any time between the beginning of September and the January deadline, most admissions tutors agree that the earlier the application is submitted, the better your chance of being called for an early round of interviews and receiving an offer.

Some universities will shortlist all applications received before 15 January but others will make offers as they go along so that by this date you may find that they have made most of their offers. The answer is to balance a really good application with getting it in near the start of the process.

If you are an Access student, this means applying very soon after you have started your course, so it may be possible to send additional information directly to the university to back up your application if necessary. Check with individual universities.

The following advice from admissions tutors illustrates the importance of an early application:

> Nursing has a high number of applicants and only suitable ones are shortlisted and interviewed. We can only make so many offers so the earlier the person makes an application, the better the chance of a place.
>
> Sally Morey, admissions tutor for adult nursing
> at Oxford Brookes University

> We start interviewing in November and we make offers as we complete each interview. We interview right through to the end of February, beginning of March. If we've made all our offers, we might be interviewing people on the understanding that if they are successful we can't make them an offer but give them an option to go on a waiting list. This only applies to people who have not got an offer elsewhere or have only applied to Oxford Brookes. So there is definitely an advantage in applying early.
>
> Heather Bower, Lead Midwife for Education
> at Oxford Brookes University

Some courses have both autumn and spring start dates. For courses that start between January and May, you should contact individual universities for advice on when to apply.

The safest bet for getting your application completed and sent as soon as possible is to make a start on it in your AS year. If you are in Scotland, you should start in the year before you start your Highers course if you aim to start university straight after completing your Highers, or in your Highers year if you aim to start university after studying for Advanced Highers.

Start researching courses and universities as early as you can and then begin writing your personal statement and get feedback on it. Ultimately, you want to be in a position where you have a final draft of your personal statement and all of your choices decided by the beginning of the September term in your A2 year or Highers/Advanced Highers year.

Suggested timescale for applications

Year 12 (fourth or fifth year of secondary education in Scotland)

It is never too early to begin to research courses and universities. Allow plenty of time for this as there will be many options to consider. Keep a check on the grades you are achieving in your coursework to inform your choice of realistic course options. Go to university open days, or nursing and midwifery taster days, as they can be useful to help you make choices between the different branches of nursing. If you don't have much relevant work experience, check whether you can get some through your school or make applications yourself: see Chapter 3 for guidance on this. You want to be in a position to be able to include in your personal statement work experience already completed and the skills and insights you have gained.

Spring: Visit university open days. Request prospectuses and departmental brochures for extra detail and look at university websites. Start work on your personal statement.

May/June: If you have missed an open day, arrange a campus visit. Continue to work on your personal statement.

June/July: Make a shortlist of your course choices before you finish for the summer break.

Year 13 (fifth or sixth year of secondary education in Scotland)

September/October/November: Complete your application online and submit it to UCAS via a referee. It can be accepted from 1 September onwards. Universities begin to make their decisions and send invitations to attend a selection day or interview. Go to any universities you have put on your application and not yet visited.

15 January: Deadline for submitting your application to UCAS.

February: If you are rejected by all of your choices, you can use UCAS Extra to look for other courses; see later in this chapter for details.

May/June: When you have received decisions from all your choices, you must tell UCAS which offer you have accepted firmly and which one is your insurance (back-up). See page 63 for more on this. You will be given a deadline by UCAS by which you must do this. Check this carefully as there are four different deadline dates depending on when you received your last decision from your university choices.

Spring: Ensure that you have completed your application for a student loan (if applicable).

Summer: Sit your exams and wait for your results. When the A level results are published, you will be able to use UCAS Track to find out whether your chosen universities have confirmed your conditional offers. If you have not got into your chosen institution, get in touch with your school/college to get help to contact the university to see whether they will still accept you. Clearing begins in mid-August, when all remaining university places are filled, but it is unlikely there will be places for nursing or midwifery at this stage. You will be sent instructions on Clearing automatically, but it is up to you to get hold of the published lists of available places and to contact the universities directly. If you have done better than expected, you can use the Adjustment system to look for universities that require higher grades, but there are unlikely to be any vacancies for nursing or midwifery at this stage.

There is further advice on what to do on results day in Chapter 9.

The reference

As well as your GCSE results and your personal statement, the admissions team will take into account your academic reference. This is usually written by your personal tutor or head of sixth form and will refer both to the grades they predict you will obtain and your suitability for the course for which you have applied. The referee is expected to be as honest as possible, and to try to accurately assess your character and potential. You may believe that you have all of the qualities – academic and personal – necessary for nursing or midwifery but unless you have demonstrated these to your teachers, they will be unable to support your application.

Make efforts to get involved in the wider life of your school or college, as well as working hard for your exams. This will help to give evidence to the people who will contribute to your reference.

As part of the reference, your referee will need to predict the grades that you are likely to achieve. Talk to your teachers and find out what these predictions are and make course choices that take this into account. It is good to aim high if this is realistic but have a few choices where the grades required are lower in case you don't do as well as expected in your exams. There is no point in applying for a course where the typical offers are higher than those you are predicted to achieve, as this is a wasted application.

Fitness to practise as a nurse or midwife

The NMC guidelines require that applicants to the NMC register need to be of good health and good character to practise as a nurse or midwife.

Good character

If you accept an offer of a place on a nursing or midwifery course, you will be asked to complete a DBS (Disclosure and Barring Service) check (formerly a CRB check) to assess that you are of good character before you can register to start the course.

On 1 December 2012, the Criminal Records Bureau (CRB) merged with the Independent Safeguarding Authority (ISA) to become The Disclosure and Barring Service (DBS). In order to work with children or vulnerable adults, it is necessary to have a DBS check (formerly a CRB check). This is a check of your police record and any criminal convictions to ensure that you are of suitable character to practise as a nurse or midwife. You will need to pay for this: the current cost for an enhanced check is £44. See www.gov.uk/crb-criminal-records-bureau-check or Disclosure Scotland, www.disclosurescotland.co.uk.

The DBS check involves completing an online application, regardless of whether you have a criminal conviction. The application asks you to disclose any convictions including spent convictions. Remember, you should always be honest and declare any convictions on your UCAS application; they may not necessarily bar you from practising as a nurse or midwife.

The information you have disclosed on your UCAS application and the results from the DBS checking process are then considered by the school of nursing/midwifery and DBS panel and an offer may be withdrawn if evidence suggests an applicant is unfit to practise, according to the NMC guidelines. If you are worried that a past conviction may bring into question your suitability for this type of work, you should contact university admissions officers for nursing and midwifery courses for advice before applying.

If you take a gap year, the DBS check will be done just before you enrol for the course.

Good health

The NMC guidelines state that to be of good health means to be capable of safe and effective practice without supervision. If you accept an offer of a place on a nursing and midwifery course, you will also be asked to complete a health-screening questionnaire, which will be assessed by the university or NHS Health Trust occupational-health department. You may be contacted by the university to discuss the information you have given or be invited to a more in-depth assessment, possibly a medical examination.

If you have any worries about being fit to practise in terms of your health, you should contact individual university admissions tutors and they may be able to give you advice or refer you to your GP for a medical examination. The NMC website (www.nmc-uk.org) also has some useful information. The NMC does not specify disabilities or health conditions that would bar a person from working as a nurse or midwife. Rather, they state on their website that 'many disabled people and those with health conditions are able to practise with or without adjustments to support their practice'. You should disclose any disabilities or health conditions; your fitness to practise will be considered on an individual basis. You should always disclose this information because the university can then guide you as to whether you can have extra help to make it possible for you to do the job. If reasonable adjustments can be made to the working environment, a person can still be fit to practise. We will look at advice for those with disabilities in Chapter 8.

Potential nursing and midwifery students also need specific inoculations (normally hepatitis B, hepatitis C, tetanus and BCG), so you should consult individual universities for further information. If you have not already had these done, they can be administered by the university occupational-health department or your GP; consult individual universities for further details.

Eligibility for NHS funding

Admission to nursing and midwifery courses is also subject to eligibility for NHS funding. Eligibility involves certain residency requirements so if you have moved to the UK in the last three years, you should check your eligibility at www.nhsbsa.nhs.uk/students. See Chapter 10 for more information.

Deferred entry

Many nursing and midwifery courses are happy to consider students who wish to take a gap year before starting their degree. However, it is very important to check with individual universities because some courses, midwifery in particular, do not accept deferred entry. Those that do may give advice on what they would expect you to do in your year off and you will need to give details of your intentions in your personal statement.

Universities will generally encourage you to gain relevant work experience to strengthen your conviction that nursing or midwifery is for you. Most important is being able to show that you are going to use the time constructively. Independent travelling, charity or voluntary work either at home or abroad, work experience or a responsible job will all indicate that you have used the time to develop independence and maturity as well as gain relevant experience. Employment as a healthcare assistant or midwifery care assistant, voluntary work abroad on a healthcare project in a developing country, work as a care assistant in a nursing home – these could all be suitable experience.

You can apply for deferred entry on your UCAS application, in which case you need to outline your plans for your gap year clearly in your personal statement. You would then receive an offer of a place before taking your year out. Equally, you could choose to apply to UCAS in the autumn after receiving your A level results, but then you would need to be available for interviews during your gap year, so this may affect your plans.

What happens next?

When you have successfully sent your UCAS application to your school or college referee (or directly to UCAS if you are applying as an individual), UCAS will send you a confirmation email to explain what happens next and will also send confirmation when your application reaches them. UCAS processes your application and sends it to each of your chosen universities and colleges and then sends you a welcome letter confirming your personal details and choices. It is vital that you check this information carefully and inform UCAS if there are any inaccuracies. Remember, you will be able to view your application at all times through the UCAS Track system using a personal ID assigned to you and the username and password that you used for Apply.

Once a university has received your application from UCAS, they may contact you to say they are considering your application; however, not all universities do this, so don't worry if you don't hear from them initially. Your prospective universities will be unable to see the other courses and universities to which you have applied.

The next stage is to wait to hear from the universities to which you applied, once they have finished considering your application. This timescale can vary enormously between universities and can be anything from a short period of time to a few months. If you are successful at the application stage, you will probably be invited to attend a selection day or interview; this information will also appear on UCAS Track so you can confirm your attendance.

We will look at what happens at selection days and interviews in Chapter 7.

After attending selection days and interviews, you will receive one of three possible responses from each university:

1. conditional offer
2. unconditional offer
3. unsuccessful application.

If you receive a conditional offer, you will be told what you need to achieve in your exams. This could be in grade terms, for example, ABB (and the university might specify a particular grade in a particular subject – ABB with a B in biology), or in UCAS Tariff points.

Unconditional offers are a straight acceptance where the student is not required to meet any conditions. These may be given to students who have already sat their A levels, such as gap-year students applying post-results.

Once you have received responses from all five universities, you will need to make your choice of the university offer you wish to accept. This is called your firm choice. You can also choose an insurance offer, effectively a second choice with a lower grade requirement. UCAS will give you a deadline by which to make this decision, so be careful to meet this deadline or you may lose your offers.

Dealing with unsuccessful applications

You may receive a notification from UCAS telling you that you have been rejected by one or more of the universities. The possible reason may appear on Track but, if not, you should contact the university to get feedback on why you were unsuccessful. If you are keen to reapply next year, you should ask for advice on how to strengthen your application.

One student voluntarily contacted us and got feedback from her interview, acted on that feedback by really taking it on board and went off and did what we had suggested. She then completely changed her personal statement and applied the next year – and was successful.

Heather Bower, Lead Midwife for Education
at Oxford Brookes University

If you show this level of commitment, occasionally universities will hold your offer at the same level. However, it is more likely that they will require you to meet the grade requirement for the following year's application cycle and may ask you to retake A levels.

UCAS Extra

If you used all your five choices on your UCAS application and have received all five decisions from UCAS and you don't have any offers, you can apply for an additional course through UCAS Extra. You can check whether courses still have vacancies by using the course search on www.ucas.com and looking for courses marked with an X. You should also contact the university directly for the most up-to-date information and to check that they are still accepting applications. Bear in mind that many nursing and midwifery courses fill up by the UCAS January deadline. UCAS Extra can be used from the end of February until early July and you can continue to apply for courses one at a time through this period if necessary.

If you still don't have any offers, you should take the opportunity to carefully reassess whether nursing or midwifery is a realistic career ambition for you and whether there were any parts of your application that let you down. If you still feel that nursing or midwifery is for you, take the opportunity to strengthen any aspects of your application that were weak. Under no circumstances should you give up and decide that it is no longer worth working hard; this will only reduce your chances of making a successful application the following year.

What to do if things go wrong during the exams

If something happens when you are preparing for, or actually taking, the exams that prevents you from doing your best, you must notify both the exam board and the universities that have made you offers. This notification will best come from your head teacher and should include your UCAS number. Send it off at once: it is no good waiting for disappointing results and then telling everyone that you were ill at the time but said nothing to anyone. Exam boards can give you special consideration if the appropriate forms are sent to them by the school, along with supporting evidence.

If you really are sufficiently ill to be unable to prepare for the exams or to perform effectively during them, you must consult your GP and obtain a letter describing your condition.

The other main cause of underperformance is distressing events at home. For example, if a member of your immediate family is seriously ill, you should explain this to your head teacher and ask them to write to the exam board and universities.

6 | Personal statement

The personal statement is one of the most important sections of the UCAS application. This is where you have the chance to tell universities your reasons for applying to, and suitability for, a particular course. You need to demonstrate your interest and commitment to nursing or midwifery and make sure that you provide a positive picture of your motivations, experiences and skills.

In this chapter we will look at how to construct a personal statement, the points it should cover and tips on how to present this information. Comments from admissions tutors on what they want to see will be used to guide you.

UCAS uses verification checks to detect copied parts of personal statements and will alert universities if they have reason to believe that you have not written your own personal statement, so do not be tempted to use sample personal statements you may find on the internet. Your personal statement should be personal to you and, above all else, it should be honest. Universities can see through students who have just followed a formula or been given a rigid structure to follow by their school or college and you are less likely to stand out from the crowd if you follow the same structure as everyone else.

TIP

The message from admissions tutors for nursing and midwifery is that they want to read an applicant's unique reasons for wanting to do nursing or midwifery and evidence of how they have come to that decision.

Remember that there is no right or wrong way to write a personal statement; you just need to ensure that it covers all the necessary points (as detailed later in this chapter) and that it gives a positive message as to why a university should consider you for a course, with the aim of getting you to the next stage – a selection day or interview.

What admissions tutors look for

Before you start writing your personal statement, put yourself in the shoes of the university admissions tutor who is going to read it. They will have a large stack of these to read so you want to ensure that you get their attention immediately and that it is interesting, easy to read, with points made clearly, and that you stand out from the crowd.

The title *personal* statement is apt. Universities are looking for more than just qualifications; they are looking for the whole person: motivations, qualities, strengths and transferable skills. Ensure that your personal statement shows why you personally want to do nursing or midwifery and it is not just a series of statements about the job and skills required. Let your personality show through what you write.

The following advice from admissions tutors will help you have a better understanding of what they are looking for:

> *We try to look for the whole person, because nursing is much more than qualifications and grades . . . what you want to see is the real person and their motivations for nursing, qualities, strengths and transferable skills and that they have an insight into adult nursing and most importantly the core values required to be an excellent healthcare professional. Anyone who applies but doesn't really show they have an idea of what adult nursing is all about and the values required, won't get shortlisted.*
>
> Sally Morey, admissions tutor for adult nursing
> at Oxford Brookes University

> *We look for an understanding and commitment to midwifery, a realistic attitude to how today's maternity care works . . . transferable skills, such as communication, leadership and working in a team . . . an understanding of diversity – childbearing women cover the whole spectrum of society . . . demonstration of a non-discriminatory attitude . . . work experience, knowledge of current issues in midwifery . . . and that they can show us what makes them stand out as an applicant.*
>
> Heather Bower, Lead Midwife for Education
> at Oxford Brookes University

> *We look for a passion for the subject, work experience, background reading – not just school biology textbooks – and outside interests.*
>
> Fiona Bazoglu, admissions officer for nursing
> at the University of Edinburgh

You should check what each individual university is looking for in terms of personal qualities, skills and work experience, and ensure that you demonstrate that you have these. Use the course search on the UCAS website to locate individual courses and their requirements; they will often state the work experience and skills they are seeking. You will also find detailed entry requirements on university websites and prospectuses.

The information that follows from the University of Manchester is fairly typical of the advice you can find on university websites on what they are expecting to see.

What information should I include in my UCAS personal statement?

Be honest about yourself when completing the personal statement. It is acceptable to write about situations where you did not achieve as well as you hoped, as you can indicate what you have learnt from the experience. If you have previously studied on nursing or other healthcare courses but did not complete the programme, please tell us as this will have been part of your personal development. You should be totally honest about declaring any previous convictions or cautions no matter how long ago or how minor the offences. Declaration will not affect your application at this stage but later identification of undeclared issues may do so.

Be accurate in relation to your academic qualifications. We ask to see original certificates or other evidence of these achievements before we offer a place. We recommend that you apply for copies of any lost documents.

Be careful as you complete your form. We receive thousands of application forms and read them all with due care and attention. Any application that is incomplete, written in poor English or contains errors will not be considered.

In order for us to consider your application and recommend that you attend for interview, your personal statement must make reference to the following areas:

- a sound rationale for your choice of nursing and particular field (adult, child or mental health)
- a summary of how your academic learning so far will help you to study in higher education (for example, time-management skills, subjects etc.)
- a statement about work-related skills (gained through either paid employment or voluntary work) demonstrating the experiences you have had which could be transferable to a career in nursing (for example, dealing with the public, customer service etc.). Please note that it is important that you detail the skills you have acquired (for example, specific communication skills)
- an understanding of and an ability to appreciate the needs of others (for example, supporting peers, understanding cultural differences).

Source: www.nursing.manchester.ac.uk/undergraduate/bnursadult/?code=07870&pg=4

Structure and content of your personal statement

When constructing your personal statement, there are several important things that you need to consider. First, your personal statement can be no more than 47 lines or 4,000 characters including spaces, to fit the allocated space on the UCAS application. You are advised to write your personal statement in a Word document, so you can check spellings and grammar and fully edit it before pasting it into the allocated space.

Second, you need to ensure that your statement addresses the following points:

- why you want to be a nurse or midwife
- your motivations for studying a particular course, e.g. adult nursing or midwifery
- your academic interests – how your A levels or equivalent qualifications will help you study in higher education and link with and support your career ambitions
- your understanding of what nursing or midwifery involves, gained through work experience and having done some research
- what you have done to develop the skills needed to become a nurse or midwife, from work experience or study
- evidence that you have the values and personal qualities needed to be a nurse or midwife
- details of your future plans and ambitions.

Follow these three steps to show that you have the experience, skills and qualities that universities are looking for.

1. Identify your skills, experience and qualities.
2. Give an example where you have personally demonstrated them.
3. Show how the experience is relevant to nursing or midwifery.

If you follow this general guideline, you will end up with a relevant, personal and insightful personal statement that will give admissions tutors the evidence they need to consider you.

Why you want to be a nurse or midwife

A high proportion of UCAS applications contain stock phrases such as: 'From an early age I have wanted to be a nurse/midwife because it combines my love of science with the chance to work with people.' Not only do admissions tutors get bored with reading such statements, but also remarks like these don't go far enough to show your personal motivations. If you think about it, there are many careers that combine science and working with people, including teaching, pharmacy, physiotherapy and medicine. It is much better to mention an incident that first got you interested in nursing, such as a hospital visit, a conversation with a family friend, a biology project or work experience where you had a taste of a caring role. Then perhaps follow this up with details of how you have pursued this interest and learnt about what the role of nurse or midwife entails by work experience and background reading.

Your motivations for studying a particular course, e.g. adult nursing

As previous chapters in the book have demonstrated, the various branches of nursing and midwifery practice are very different. The admissions team reviewing your application will expect to see your whole application directed towards midwifery or a specific branch of nursing. This is where it is very important for you to have made a decision about the branch of nursing that you want to study and that all five of your choices are for this branch. If you apply for more than one area of nursing, the result will be an unfocused personal statement or one that just highlights that you are undecided.

> If they apply for a whole range of nursing fields, their statement becomes too general and they won't be shortlisted. They need to have done their preparation before they apply, by going to open days and speaking to tutors from the different nursing branches . . . they need to know what they want to do and why they want to do it.
>
> Sally Morey, admissions tutor for adult nursing at Oxford Brookes University

Your academic interests

Show that you are interested in and able to study for three years at degree level. You need to show that you have researched the course and know what it will involve. Mention both the university-based study and the placements, perhaps referring to specific modules you have seen in course descriptions. Mention skills and experiences you have that will help you succeed on the course and how your current studies relate to the course.

Your understanding of what nursing/midwifery involves

It is important to back up evidence of your initial interest in nursing/ midwifery with details of what you have done to investigate the career both in terms of work experience and research.

This is where you can describe your work experience. It is important to demonstrate that you gained something from the work experience and that it has given you an insight into the profession. You should give an indication of the length of time you spent on work experience, what you observed, and impressions you've gained of the different areas of nursing. You could comment on the aspects of the particular branch you are applying to that attract you, what you found interesting or something that you hadn't expected. Beyond this, you should also mention any other work experience you have had in a caring role or where you have gained relevant skills.

Here is a sample description of a student's work experience that would probably not impress the admissions team.

I spent a week at a nursing home talking to patients and observing nurses and care assistants.

In contrast, the following example would be much more convincing because it is clear that the student is interested in what was happening.

During my two weeks at a care home, I helped the care assistants talk to patients, serve meals and run activities for the elderly residents. I was also able to watch a qualified nurse give an injection and administer medicines and I helped calculate the dosage. I was able to develop my communication skills by talking to residents with a range of conditions, including dementia, and realised how important it is to listen. I enjoyed making sure patients were comfortable and happy and at the end of the week felt certain that a caring role is for me. A number of things surprised me: in particular, how demanding and tiring it can be, but also how satisfying.

It will be far easier to write this section of your personal statement if you spent some time making notes during your work experience. Look back over what you wrote and use your thoughts and experiences as information for this section.

If you are a mature student, you will probably have more work experience, so make sure that you expand on this and the skills gained relevant to nursing and midwifery. It is not enough just to list jobs in the Employment section of the UCAS application.

Show understanding of, and commitment to, nursing or midwifery. Common mistakes are to say 'I love babies' or 'I've had my own family' as a reason for wanting to do midwifery, which signals a lack of understanding of the job. The role is much more about supporting women, so you should give examples of work experience where you have worked with a range of women. Show that you understand all aspects of the role.

You also need to demonstrate a realistic attitude to nursing or midwifery, an understanding of how today's healthcare works, gained from talking to qualified practitioners and reading relevant newspaper articles, journals and websites. Refer to Chapter 7 for more help with issues you should be aware of and useful sources of information. Try to find an interesting but different relevant article to make you stand out from the crowd.

Show you have relevant values and personal qualities

The person reading your UCAS application has to decide whether you have the right skills and personal qualities to become a successful nurse or midwife, such as communication skills, teamworking and leadership, organisational skills, working with a diverse range of people and ability to understand and appreciate the needs of others. Don't just mention that you have communication skills; give personal examples of where you developed them and then show how they are transferable and apply them to nursing or midwifery.

You should give lots of evidence of how you have demonstrated and developed these qualities. Evidence doesn't need to just come from nursing, midwifery and care experience. Working in retail, catering, customer services or any jobs working with the public can give you transferable skills. You need to identify these and show how they are going to be valuable to nursing or midwifery. Skills can be gained from positions of responsibility in and out of school, being a peer mentor, being a member or captain of a sports team, activities in preparation for higher education such as taster days, taking part in the Duke of Edinburgh Scheme or other ways of demonstrating that you are able to work in teams or show leadership. If you have any unusual interests or take part in unusual activities, these can make you stand out, especially if you can show that skills gained from these are transferable to nursing or midwifery.

You need to be able to demonstrate that you have made efforts to participate in a range of worthwhile activities and that you are a well-rounded person.

Writing style

Use solid examples, not vague statements. Avoid statements that are common knowledge; don't tell admissions tutors what they already know! For example:

Nursing is a very demanding yet rewarding job.

This says nothing about your personal experiences of the challenges of nursing. Instead, give an example of a situation where you found out that nursing is demanding, such as trying to communicate with someone with dementia or observing a busy hospital ward. Show why you feel it would be rewarding, for example, from your experiences of talking to a midwife about why they like their job, or of voluntary work you may have done, such as helping someone with a learning disability go shopping.

Don't be too informal and try to use professional language to demonstrate that you have some understanding of current nursing and midwifery issues. You may find the glossary at the end of the book useful.

Once the personal statement is complete

When you have completed your personal statement you must ensure that you check it for any spelling and grammatical errors. You may find it easier to print out the personal statement, as it is easier to spot mistakes from a printed version than on a screen.

Finally, ask yourself: does the personal statement really reflect who you are? Will the university admissions staff who read it feel the passion and interest that you have for nursing or midwifery? Ask someone whose opinion you trust and who will be objective to review what you have written.

You will finally need to paste it into your UCAS application, ensuring that it is the right length (see page 68).

7 | Selection days

This chapter will cover university selection days, what they may involve and suggestions on how you can best prepare for them. You will find tips on interview technique and suggestions on how to tackle typical interview questions. We will also look at the group activities you may encounter, such as group interviews and discussions. Tips from admissions tutors, and one student's experiences of two very different selection days, will give you an insight into what to expect.

What to expect

Selection days can be a half day to a full day. They may include:

- presentation about the course and university
- tour of campus
- individual interview
- group interview
- group discussion or activity, which will sometimes lead to giving a presentation
- English test
- maths test
- chance to ask current nursing/midwifery students questions.

Universities use selection days to find out first-hand whether the impression you gave on your UCAS application and personal statement is accurate, and to investigate your suitability for their course and for the role of nurse or midwife. They may have a grading system to decide to whom they make offers and may grade you on your UCAS application, individual interview, group activity and tests, as well as their general impressions of you throughout the day.

> We observe them throughout the day, see how they interact, work with others and assess whether what we see in the group activity and interview measure up with what we have read in their personal statement. We can pick out people who haven't written their own statement, or who haven't done their preparation or have applied for nursing for the wrong reasons.
>
> Sally Morey, admissions tutor for adult nursing
> at Oxford Brookes University

Admissions tutors may use a screening tool (a list of attributes and knowledge they are looking for) to measure the suitability of each applicant.

This is an example screening tool for midwifery:

- knowledge about midwifery
- motivation to midwifery
- communication skills, compassion, empathy
- able to work in a team
- able to be non-judgemental, knows importance of inclusion and values diversity
- able to be flexible, considers alternatives
- self-confidence and potential to instil confidence in women and families
- has prepared for interview, shows knowledge and has questions to ask
- academic writing skills.

Universities change their selection procedures regularly and it is important to look at individual university websites and prospectuses for information (if any) about what a selection day may involve.

Planning ahead

Check all the information you have received from the university so that you know exactly where and when you will need to be on the day. Ensure that you sort out your travel arrangements so that you arrive on time and dress smartly.

Throughout the day, be polite, attentive and positive. Enjoy the day and try not to worry about nerves – admissions staff know that candidates will be nervous and will bear this in mind when making their decisions, but if you clam up completely they will be unable to assess your suitability for the course. Try to have your say, listen to others and contribute without dominating.

Interviews

Most nursing and midwifery courses conduct face-to-face individual interviews as part of their assessment process. These may be as short as 10 minutes, with only a short time in which to make a good impression. The interview will probably be carried out by a panel of at least two people, which can include university staff, practising nurses or midwives or even service users (clients or patients who receive nursing or midwifery services).

Confidence at interview comes from being prepared. Start by keeping a folder with a printout of your UCAS form and personal statement. Keep the university prospectus and any information about the course that you have been given and make a collection of articles about current issues in nursing or midwifery that you have read in national newspapers, journals or on websites. Practise answering some typical questions asked at interview (see later in the chapter) and make sure that you have written down some questions you could ask. Study your folder before the day to ensure that you are fully prepared.

In any interview situation, it makes a better impression if you arrive in plenty of time for your interview and dress smartly and appropriately. Initial impressions are very important. Remember that if the interviewers cannot picture you as a nurse or midwife in the future, they are unlikely to offer you a place. Try to appear confident and enthusiastic in your interview – but listen carefully to the questions you are asked without interrupting, and always answer honestly.

Interview questions

Interview questions are designed to find out how interested you are and motivated to study nursing or midwifery and your suitability for the course and eventual job roles. Questions are likely to test your knowledge of nursing and midwifery and developments in healthcare. Any nursing or midwifery topics that have recently been in the news could well be interview topics and you should be informed enough to have an opinion about them.

It is important that your answers are delivered in appropriate language. You will impress interviewers with some knowledge of terminology relating to nursing and midwifery. You may find it useful to refer to the glossary at the end of the book for some of the words and phrases you should know.

You might be asked which part of your A level courses (or equivalent) you have most enjoyed. You need to think carefully before your interview whether any parts of your courses relate well to nursing, midwifery or healthcare. Subjects such as human biology, sociology or psychology, or health and social care could all include relevant topics you could mention.

You will almost certainly be asked about any relevant work experience, so you should think about specific tasks and experiences where you have learnt about the role of nurse or midwife.

Don't forget that interview skills are greatly improved by practice. Try to arrange for a careers adviser, teacher or family friend to give you a mock interview.

Typical interview questions

The following are typical questions you may be asked with suggestions as to how you should go about answering them. Admissions tutors will vary the wording of questions they ask but they tend to fall into the main topic areas that follow. Remember, universities are not looking for model answers but want to find out about you, your values, attributes, personality and knowledge of nursing or midwifery. Ensure that your answer is personal to you, positive but also honest.

Question: Tell me why you decided to apply to this university

The interviewers will be looking for evidence of research about their particular course and university. Probably the best possible answer would start with 'I came to your open day . . .' because you can then proceed to tell them why you like their university, what impressed you about the course and facilities and how the atmosphere of the place would particularly suit you. If you were unable to attend an open day, try to arrange a formal or informal visit before you are interviewed so that you can show that you are aware of the environment and that it would suit you. It is vital to do your homework by reading the prospectus and looking at the university website. Although on the surface all courses in each field of nursing appear to cover broadly the same subjects, there are big differences between the ways in which courses are delivered and in the opportunities for patient contact, and your interviewers will expect you to know about their course.

Possible answer: 'I came to an open day last summer, which is why I have applied here. I enjoyed the day, and was impressed by the facilities and the comments of the students who showed us around, because they seemed so enthusiastic about the course. Also, I really like the wide choice of community-based placements and the possibility of an elective placement abroad in the third year.'

Question: What attracted you to nursing/midwifery?

This is the question that all applicants expect. Since 'Why do you want to be a nurse?' is such an obvious question, interviewers often try to find out the information in different ways. Expect questions such as 'When did your interest in nursing start?', or 'What was it about your work experience that finally convinced you that nursing was for you?'

Given that the interviewers will be aware that you are expecting the question, they will also expect your answer to be carefully planned. If you look surprised and say something like 'Um . . . well . . . I haven't really thought about why . . .', you can expect to be rejected.

Many students are worried that they will sound insincere when they answer this question. The way to avoid this is to try to bring in reasons that are personal to you: for example, an incident that sparked your interest, perhaps being inspired by nurses at a visit to a hospital, or an aspect of your work experience that attracted you to nursing or mid-wifery. The important thing is to try to express clearly what interested you instead of generalising your answers. Rather than saying 'nursing combines science and caring for people' – which says little about you – tell the interviewers what sparked off your interest in nursing or midwifery.

Possible answer: 'It was when I did my second work experience, which was at a nursing home, that I decided nursing was for me. I had previously spent a week at a care home, spending time with the elderly residents, sharing activities and making sure that they were comfortable, and found out that I really enjoy the care role. My second work experience was at a nursing home where the patients all needed medical care from a nursing team. Here I was able to observe nurses using clinical skills, as well as caring for patients, and I decided I wanted to learn these skills. My mum's friend is a nurse, so I talked to her and she told me about the harder parts of the job but that she found it very satisfying. When I came to your nursing information day I found out about the topics I would learn on a degree and the sorts of placements I would do and this really confirmed for me that nursing is what I want to do.'

Question: What is the role of a nurse/midwife?
There are a range of possible questions closely related to this one, aiming to investigate your general understanding of nursing and midwifery and more specifically about the branch of nursing for which you are applying. It is probably best to use an example from work experience to show how you have a personal insight, either from observing or trying things yourself. Try to show that you understand some of the skills needed, such as communication skills, teamworking and being organised.

Question: Why are you interested in the particular course that you have applied for?
This question gives you the chance to show that you have made an informed decision about the branch of nursing for which you are applying, perhaps by mentioning any relevant work experience that helped you confirm your choice of branch, or a visit to an open day where you found out about the different branches. Show why you have chosen this particular course and how it differs from other nursing courses.

Question: What relevant work experience do you have?
This could include both directly relevant work experience, such as in a hospital, care home or for a charity, as well as voluntary work or employment where you have been able to develop skills that you could apply to nursing, such as communication skills, organisation skills, teamworking and leadership. Remember that all work experience is valuable as long as you can demonstrate the transferable skills you have gained and how they are relevant to nursing or midwifery.

Question: I see that you spent two weeks doing a placement in a hospital. Was there anything that surprised you?

Variations on this question could include 'Was there anything that particularly interested you?', 'Was there anything you found off-putting?' or simply 'Tell me about your work experience'. What these questions are really asking are whether you are able to show that you were interested in what was happening during your work experience and that you got a realistic picture and made a decision on whether it was for you based on a real insight.

Saying 'Yes, I was surprised by the number of patients who seemed very scared' sounds as if it was a negative experience for you. However, answering 'Yes, I was surprised by the number of patients who seemed very scared. What struck me, however, was the way in which the nurse dealt with each patient as an individual, sometimes being sympathetic, sometimes explaining things in great detail and sometimes using humour to relax them' shows that you were interested enough to be aware of how nurses dealt with this.

Question: Tell us about a health-related article you have read recently.

If you are interested in making nursing or midwifery your career, the selectors will expect you to be interested enough in the subject to want to read about it. Some good sources of information that you may want to use are:

- NHS: www.nhs.uk (has a section on health news)
- Department of Health: www.dh.gov.uk
- BBC News: www.bbc.co.uk/news/health
- Royal College of Nursing: www.rcn.org.uk and http://thisisnursing. rcn.org.uk
- *Nursing Standard* (journal from the RCN): www.nursingstandard. rcnpublishing.co.uk
- *Nursing Times*: www.nursingtimes.net (you need to subscribe to access all the content)
- Royal College of Midwives: www.rcm.org.uk
- *Midwives* (journal from the RCM): www.rcm.org.uk/midwives
- www.studentmidwife.net.

You should also get into the habit of checking the news every day to see whether there are any nursing-related or midwifery-related stories. See the section later in this chapter on current issues in nursing and midwifery.

Question: How will you cope with the academic demands of the course?

Admissions tutors want to be sure that you are aware of the demands of doing a three-year degree including a dissertation. You could talk about your current A levels (or equivalent) and how you have enjoyed particular topics (choose ones that relate to nursing or midwifery) and how you are keen to develop this knowledge further. Talk about group projects or your involvement in any presentations and your approach to independent learning, to show that you welcome study at this level.

Other possible questions

Here are a selection of questions that have been asked in university interviews for nursing or midwifery courses. You can use these as a basis for a mock interview. Ask someone who does not know you very well to ask you a selection of relevant questions from the list, and then ask them to assess how convincing your answers were. If there are areas that are obviously in need of work, then you can do some further research in preparation for the real interview.

- What do you think makes a good nurse/midwife?
- What specific qualities do you have to make an effective nurse/midwife?
- What sort of person are you? (**hint** – include reliable, good communicator, organised, able to work both independently and in a team etc. and provide examples to show that you have these qualities.)
- Where does nursing take place? (**hint** – not just in hospitals – also in the community, patients' homes etc.)
- What skills make you suitable for this course?
- How prepared are you for university – what is going to be your biggest challenge?
- What would friends say are your good and bad points? (**hint** – concentrate on the positive points.)
- How will you manage your time on the course?
- Give an example of when you have dealt with a traumatic situation.
- How would you cope with the death of a patient?
- Why are good communication skills important for the role of nurse/midwife?
- What does confidentiality mean and why is it important?
- How would you deal with a difficult patient? (**hint** – show you can be non-judgemental.)
- Imagine you are a nurse on a ward/midwife in the community, what could you be doing?
- What do you think patients feel like in A&E?
- What do you know about the NMC?
- How would you deal with a team member you disagree with?
- You are walking down a ward and see a patient struggling to get dressed. What do you do?
- What is evidence-based care?

Current issues in nursing and midwifery

It is essential to have a good understanding of current issues in the world of nursing and midwifery. Here are a few topics you may be asked about, as a starting point for you to do further research.

Rise in long-term health conditions

Advances in treatment mean that more people are now surviving ill-nesses that would have limited their life expectancy in the past. This means that there are now many more people living in the community with a long-term health condition that, although serious, is not immedi-ately life-threatening but needs continuing care. These conditions include diabetes, asthma, chronic obstructive pulmonary disease (COPD), coronary heart disease, epilepsy, arthritis and cancer. Accord-ing to the Department of Health, there are around 15 million people in England with at least one long-term condition, a condition that cannot be cured but can be managed through medication and/or therapy.

This has resulted in more nurses working in the community, to support people as far as possible to manage these conditions in their own homes and to reduce the need to go into hospital. Hospitals are increas-ingly considered to be places for people who are very unwell who need more complex treatment or investigations. Nurses are involved in pro-viding services and producing personalised care plans to help individu-als manage long-term conditions. This can include systems to allow people with long-term conditions to have control over their own care, such as Telehealth, using electronic sensors or equipment that monitors vital health signs remotely, in a person's own home or on the move. The results of this can be monitored by a healthcare professional who can decide whether to intervene, without a patient needing to attend a clinic. This has been shown to reduce hospital admissions. All nurses and midwives have a duty to provide health education as part of their role, in relation to topics such as smoking and weight management, to minimise the onset of conditions such as COPD and heart disease.

NHS cuts and reorganisation

It is important to show that you have a realistic view of the challenges of being a nurse or midwife in the current economic climate. Although the government pledged to protect front-line jobs and that cuts would be mostly at managerial level, NHS Information Centre figures show that there has been a loss of more than 6,000 qualified-nursing posts and a corresponding reduction of places on university courses. However, in many Health Trusts, savings are being made in other ways to avoid cut-ting nursing posts, so consult the website for your local Health Trust for the situation in your local area and ask your local university for employment rates for nursing and midwifery courses. The number of midwives being recruited is slowly increasing.

Some hospital departments have been closed in favour of services being concentrated in bigger and better-staffed hospitals. This has resulted, in some areas, in fewer local services and more need to travel for treatment. Nurses now work in multidisciplinary teams and in partnership with other services, such as social services. Hospitals are now more for the very sick, with other people being looked after in the community or at home. Clinical-commissioning groups, formed by groups of GP practices, are beginning to have responsibility for planning and delivery of healthcare and this may have an impact on nursing in the future.

Dementia care

According to the Department of Health, about 750,000 people in the UK have dementia and this number is expected to double in the next 30 years. There has been an increase in funding for dementia research and for care homes and hospitals to create special areas for people with dementia to help reduce patient anxiety and stress. There is also increased support for healthcare professionals to spot dementia, including resources for nurses following the SPACE principles:

- **S**killed staff
- **P**artnership with carers
- **A**ssessment and early identification
- **C**are that is individualised
- **E**nvironments that are dementia friendly.

Learning to care for patients with dementia, both in hospitals and the community, will be an important focus for nursing in the future.

MRSA

This is a type of bacterial infection that is resistant to a number of antibiotics and can lead to life-threatening infections. Infection rates have fallen significantly in recent years but over 6% of hospital patients in England still acquire some sort of infection during their stay, according to the Health Protection Agency (HPA). MRSA infections are more common in hospitals and nursing homes where there are a large number of ill or vulnerable people together and where bacteria can more easily spread, and because patients with wounds have an entry point for bacteria. It is important that nurses and midwives are aware of this and can take precautions such as frequent hand washing.

Elective Caesareans

Midwifery applicants should be aware of the debate about healthy women asking for elective Caesareans and whether this is appropriate just for 'social convenience'. Some say that all women should be given support, information and possibly referred for counselling and then, if after counselling they still don't want a natural birth, they should have the option of a Caesarean. Others would only make exceptions for those who have had a difficult or traumatic birth previously, or who have mental-health issues. There is also the opinion that midwives should help women overcome their fear of childbirth. See the NHS Choices website for more information, www.nhs.uk.

Other topics you could research are healthy eating in pregnancy, the importance of health promotion as part of the role of nurse/midwife, whether all women should breastfeed, the increase in community nurses and the increase in mental-health problems.

Group interview

Owing to the large number of applicants, some universities may not offer you an individual interview. Instead, you may be interviewed in a small group, where each person is asked the same question in turn. The questions can be very similar to those asked in an individual interview and can include questions about reasons for choosing nursing or midwifery, the course, the university, skills needed for nursing or midwifery, relevant healthcare topics and difficult scenarios you may encounter, such as a patient with communication problems. As the interview proceeds, interviewers may vary the order in which questions are asked or candidates may be picked at random to answer. You should prepare for this in much the same way as for an individual interview but make sure that you have prepared several different answers to more typical questions, as someone might give the answer you were going to give!

Interview checklist

Before the interview

- Find out about the interview format, whether you will have an individual or group interview, how many people will be on the interview panel, so that you can prepare appropriately.
- Look at the information that you provided about yourself on your UCAS application and personal statement and be prepared to answer questions, clarify, or expand on any of this.
- Make sure that you have read the course details in both the university prospectus and on the website and ensure that you are familiar

with the course and what makes it different from courses at other universities. Ensure that you have good reasons for choosing the course and that you have prepared some questions you genuinely want to ask (not covered by information in the university website/prospectus).

- Refer back to articles about current issues in nursing or midwifery that you have read in national newspapers, journals or on websites and have a few topics in mind you could talk about in the interview.
- Prepare specific positive points about yourself you want to come across in the interview.
- Write down possible answers to a range of common questions.
- Use chat forums to speak to others who have had interviews, to learn from their experiences.
- Plan your journey, take a map of the campus, allow enough time to arrive early and find the room in plenty of time.
- Take the phone number of the appropriate university admissions department in case you have to ring to say that you are delayed.
- Turn off your mobile before you go into your interview!

Body language

- Maintain eye contact with the interviewers, smile.
- Direct most of what you are saying to the person who asked you the question, but also acknowledge the reactions of other interviewers.
- Sit up straight, but adopt a position that is comfortable for you.

Speech

- Take time to think about what you want to say and try to talk slowly and clearly.
- Listen to the question carefully so that you give a relevant answer, not just what you want to say.
- Be enthusiastic about the course and university.
- Don't be too informal, have a professional bearing.
- Don't be afraid to ask for a question to be repeated, to give yourself more time to think of an answer and be honest if you don't understand the question or don't know the answer.
- Avoid one-word answers, like yes and no, the interviewer needs to know enough about you to make a decision.
- Remember that it is a two-way process, you also need to find out whether the course is right for you, so ask about any aspects of the course where you need clarification.

Dress and appearance

- Wear clothes that show that you have made an effort for the interview. Dress smartly but comfortably, suitable for the day's activities.
- Make sure that you are clean and tidy.

After the interview

- Reflect on the experience, did you feel comfortable with the process, like the interviewers, the environment?
- Write down the questions you were asked (and your replies, if you can remember), this will be useful for future interviews.

If you are unsuccessful in receiving an offer of a place, you may be given feedback straight away. Try to remain positive and make sure that you write down what you would need to do to boost your application or improve your performance, should you decide to reapply at a later date.

Reasons for unsuccessful interviews

A main reason given by admissions tutors for applicants not being successful at interview is giving a superficial answer without depth or a model answer they have read somewhere.

> *Sometimes we can see they are not really thinking beyond the surface about anything, they haven't really engaged with what midwifery is or what the issues are.*
>
> Heather Bower, Lead Midwife for Education
> at Oxford Brookes University

Another reason for applicants being unsuccessful, according to admissions staff, is where an applicant assumes that they already have the knowledge they need; for example, if they have worked as a maternity care assistant or healthcare assistant or have had their own children, they think that they automatically have the experience and knowledge they need to train to be a nurse or midwife. The admissions tutor would then question the applicant further, to check whether they have a clear idea about the differences between working in an assistant role and being a nurse or midwife.

Other reasons quoted for applicants being unsuccessful include having an unrealistic view of the role of midwife or nurse; and applicants not conducting themselves in a professional manner at interview, being too informal or being too detached. Bear in mind that the interviewer needs to imagine you as a nurse or midwife, showing warmth and compassion in human interactions and with a professional approach.

Group discussion or activity

If you are not given a group interview, you can expect some type of group activity, as admissions tutors will want to see how you interact with others. You may be put in small groups and asked to discuss specified topics. These topics will probably be ones that allow admissions tutors to assess your opinions as well as your background knowledge.

We tend to focus on topics which allow the applicants to explore values and attitudes as well as knowledge. These may include current issues in healthcare and the related choices a woman may make, such as the choice to have an elective Caesarean section or whether or not to breastfeed her baby.

Luisa Acosta, Senior Midwifery Lecturer and Admissions Co-ordinator at the University of West London

You need to be confident enough to put your view across, but equally to listen to and appreciate other applicants' points of view and to comment and expand on these. It is important to find a balance between contributing and not dominating. The interviewing staff may move back and observe from the sidelines to allow the discussion to flow freely, but remember that they will be listening to each individual's contribution and making decisions based on this.

You may be given a prioritisation activity, for example, where you have case studies of four patients and are told that you only have time to see two and, as a group, have to decide which two you would choose to see and why. In this exercise the admissions tutors are not looking so much for background knowledge, but rather as to how you integrate and negotiate with other applicants.

Sometimes they will ask the group to present the conclusions of their discussion. Again, admissions staff will be looking to see who takes the lead with this, who is a good facilitator, who is good at listening to everyone's views and so on. Generally, they want to see that you could work well in groups, both on the course and in a future teamwork role, and that you have the appropriate communication skills, attitudes and values for nursing or midwifery.

We hold group interviews where candidates work in groups with an on-course student. They are asked to prepare a presentation 'What is nursing?' – which they present to the other candidates. They are encouraged to be creative in their presentation and communicate between themselves.

Fiona Bazoglu, admissions officer for nursing at the University of Edinburgh

English and maths tests

You may be asked to sit a short test in English or maths as part of a selection day. The NMC sets literacy and numeracy guidelines and it is up to universities to ensure that they make offers to applicants who will be able to cope with the academic demands of the course and who by the end of the course have literacy and numeracy skills at an adequate standard to register as a qualified nurse or midwife.

Some universities no longer use English and maths tests as they set specific GCSE English and maths entry requirements (or equivalent) and feel that this gives them enough information about an applicant's ability to cope with the demands of the course, but others will set tests as part of the selection day.

English (literacy) tests

Tests can differ widely and are designed both to check that you have the skills needed to study at degree level and to assess whether you would be able to cope with the academic demands of the course. You could be asked questions that test your comprehension of an article relating to healthcare, nursing or midwifery or be given a topic and asked to write a short essay or prepare a short presentation to give to other applicants. The exercise could include reflecting on an experience, how it has affected you and what you have learnt from it, and then writing about it.

Maths (numeracy) tests

The NMC sets guidelines that potential nurses and midwives need to be able to do addition, subtraction, multiplication, division, averages, percentages, fractions, ratios, converting millilitres to litres, and seconds to minutes, and decimal places. Confidence with these sorts of maths skills is vital in the job to calculate correct dosages of medication and measure patients' temperature, fluid intake etc. Questions may include realistic scenarios, such as for midwifery, calculating a drug dose for a baby of a particular weight. As well as your old GCSE maths notes, the BBC skillswise site may be useful for revision, www.bbc.co.uk/skillswise.

Some universities purely use tests to see whether a potential student will need extra help with English or maths on the course. Some universities put sample tests on their website with answers. At some universities you may have to pass the tests to progress to the interview stage.

If you are adequately prepared, selection days should give you the chance to expand on what you have demonstrated in your personal statement – that you have fully considered and understood the nursing or midwifery role you have applied for and have the skills and personal qualities to make an effective nurse or midwife.

One student's experiences of selection days

Holly went to several selection days for midwifery courses; her experiences of two of them may help you prepare.

There were only seven of us on the selection day. It started with a presentation about the university and the midwifery degree. We then sat in a circle and were invited to ask a student midwife questions about the course or life at university. It was difficult to think of questions because the presentation had covered most things. This was followed by a group activity where the seven of us sat round a table with paper and pens and were asked as a group to prepare a presentation on healthy eating in pregnancy. We were told they wouldn't mark what we wrote but were more interested in how we worked as a team and discussed the issues. Some people were very dominant and it was difficult to get a word in edgeways and consequently I think I came across as shy when I am not! This was then followed by a 20-minute individual interview. Unfortunately I wasn't successful in getting an offer from this university.

I was more prepared for the next selection day I went to (for a different university) – I had thought of lots of possible questions I could ask and I made sure I didn't sit in a group with people who were very domineering. This day was very different, there were 60 of us! First we had a presentation with a chance to ask questions and then we were split into two groups, to have a maths test and a group activity. The group activity involved sitting in groups of four and discussing the role of a midwife. I was shocked to find that we weren't going to be offered an individual interview, so this activity was in effect the interview. I asked lots of questions so they would remember me and in order to make myself stand out. I received an offer of a place on this course.

Holly Janine Bexson Smith, first-year student
at De Montfort University

8 | Non-standard applications

Much of the information you will find on university websites and prospectuses is focused on standard entry requirements and application procedures for A level students, so if you are a mature student, an international student or an EU student, if English is not your first language, if you have a disability or additional needs, or if you are an overseas-trained nurse or midwife, it can be more difficult to find relevant entry information.

This chapter gives advice on the entry requirements for specific applicants, on available support to students with a disability or additional needs, and provides some of the answers to questions commonly asked by mature students. It also looks at opportunities to study abroad and, if you do so, equally at the requirements set by the NMC to practise as a nurse or midwife in the UK.

Universities usually provide some information on alternative entry requirements for pre-registration nursing and midwifery courses but if it is not clear whether the qualifications you are offering would be suitable for entry, you should contact the university admissions tutor for the course in which you are interested.

Mature students

A significant proportion of applicants to nursing and midwifery courses are mature students. In 2012, 19,708 applicants were 20 and under; 10,785 were aged 21 to 24; 18,548 were aged 25 to 39; and 4,930 were aged 40 and over. Mature applicants need to show that they would be able to cope with the academic demands of the course and universities will usually require evidence of recent study, usually at level 3 (A level or equivalent) within the last three to five years. You should check with individual universities for their specific requirements. Universities will consider much more than just your qualifications and will take into account your work and life experiences. It is also a requirement of the NMC that applicants are physically fit to practise as a nurse or midwife.

Mature students often feel that the UCAS application process is geared more towards young people and that the information universities give about entry requirements is not appropriate to them. If your qualifications are not listed or if you want to see whether your experience will offset a lack of qualifications, you should contact the individual universities. They may be able to use APL (accreditation of prior learning) to assess whether recent study can be counted towards entry requirements. APEL (accreditation of prior experiential learning) is an extension of this and includes learning from relevant life and work experience and may also count towards entry.

Many further-education colleges offer Access to Higher Education Diploma courses, specifically designed for mature students who need to update their academic skills before they apply for a degree in nursing or midwifery. See Chapter 2 for more details about Access courses. These courses are widely accepted by universities but you should check with individual institutions about the credits and grades they would expect you to get in order to make you an offer of a place.

Mature student FAQS

Will I have to work any night shifts?

Yes, students are expected to experience the full 24-hour pattern of care on placement. All students will work some early starts, late finishes, nights and weekends. However, it is frequently possible to plan shifts well in advance, for example, to accommodate occasional family events or a partner's employment pattern. It is not possible to arrange shifts around school times. You would need to take holidays at fixed times.

Will childcare facilities be available?

Probably, but you will have to plan childcare carefully as you will spend time both at university and on placement. Either of these settings may well offer childcare facilities but they may not necessarily open for early starts or late finishes. Most parents find independent arrangements are best; most areas have childminders who could be available for the variety of shifts students are expected to work on placement. Sure Start Children's Centres, www.gov.uk/find-sure-start-childrens-centre, are good sources of information on childcare options.

Is there any funding for childcare?

If you are entitled to an NHS bursary, you may be able to get some help with childcare costs. See www.nhsbsa.nhs.uk/816.aspx. You may also be eligible for a Dependants Allowance or Parent Learning Allowance, payable if you have people wholly or mainly financially dependent on you during your training, such as a spouse, partner or children.

All full-time students are usually either exempt from council tax or are entitled to discounts.

What if my children are unwell? Can I take time off?

There are fixed requirements for nursing and midwifery courses; any time missed will need to be 'made up'. However, universities should be sympathetic to your circumstances.

Will I have to travel far for placements?

This will vary according to the university but for most people there will be an element of travel to placements as you will need to do placements in a variety of settings. Check with your preferred universities. Your university may take account of your circumstances and access to transport; check carefully before you apply. If you are entitled to an NHS bursary, you may be reimbursed for some of the cost of travel to placements and accommodation costs on placement.

Will my experience as a care worker/healthcare assistant be helpful?

Yes, definitely, as you will have an insight into some of the roles and demands of working in the healthcare sector. However, you will still need to demonstrate that you can cope with the academic demands of the course. You will also have to show that you understand the differences between your current role and that of nurse or midwife and research these roles thoroughly.

Students with a disability or additional needs

If you have a disability or additional needs and are not sure whether you will meet the NMC's fitness-to-practise criteria, you should in the first instance contact the admissions tutor for the nursing or midwifery course in which you are interested. After a brief discussion, they may be able to give you advice on the spot or, alternatively, ask you for a further health report from your GP or refer you to the university occupational-health team. In order to make a decision, universities will consider the tasks that need to be done as a nurse or midwife and how your disability may affect your ability to do these tasks, looking at each potential student on an individual basis. They will look at whether a specific branch of nursing or midwifery could be a realistic option for you and whether adaptations can be made to the course and the kind of support you could expect to receive.

They may also refer you to the university disability officer or disability services who help students with sensory and mobility impairments, dyslexia and other learning difficulties, and mental-health issues. You can get advice and support on physical access, funding, alternative assessment arrangements (such as having a scribe in an exam). A disability officer can liaise with teaching staff to ensure that they are aware of your requirements.

You should always disclose a disability on your UCAS form and you can expect universities to be supportive. Consider these views from the University of Birmingham website and from an admissions tutor.

> We take a positive view of what candidates with disabilities can achieve as future healthcare professionals and take seriously our obligation to make reasonable adjustments to ensure that all students with disabilities can successfully complete their studies. All applicants will be assessed up to and including the interview on the basis of the criteria outlined above regardless of any disability. If you declare a disability we will invite you to work with us together with the disability team, clinical colleagues and specialist services to explore how best we can support your studies.
>
> Source: www.birmingham.ac.uk/students/courses/undergraduate/med/nursing.aspx#CourseDetailsTab

It's always better to be upfront about these things, because we can't make reasonable adjustments if we don't know about it . . . we can discuss the nature of the disability and look at the tasks to be done as a midwife and see if there may be an issue . . . having a disability won't necessarily prevent them from being a midwife.

Heather Bower, Lead Midwife for Education
at Oxford Brookes University

You may find it useful to look at the website of Disability Rights UK, www.disabilityrightsuk.org/disabledstudents.htm, for useful information on benefits and the types of support universities can provide.

Most universities also have a study-skills service and offer help with planning and writing essays and dissertations, research, support with maths and statistics, and preparing for exams.

International students

As the Department of Health funds the tuition fees for nursing and midwifery courses, most universities will not accept applications from students who are not eligible for NHS funding. This is due to NHS restrictions on funding and placements. If you are ordinarily resident outside the EEA (European Economic Area) you are not usually eligible for NHS funding. However, there are exceptions and you should check eligibility at www.nhsbsa.nhs.uk/Students.aspx. When there are high numbers of UK and EEA applicants and a restricted number of places available on each course, universities are often not in a position to consider non-EEA students. A small number of universities may consider non-EEA students if they can self-fund. You must check with individual universities but opportunities will be very limited.

EEA students or those with English as a second language

If you are an EEA student or if English is not your first language, you must be able to meet the English-language requirements set by individual universities for entry to pre-registration courses. The NMC gives guidance to universities that their admissions and selection criteria should include evidence of capacity to develop literacy skills to cope with the programme. In many cases universities ask for a score of 7.0 in the International English Language Test (IELTS).

Individual universities may accept you if you have TOEFL (Test of English as a Foreign Language) equivalencies or other language qualifications; or if you received most of your education in English; or if you have a degree in English language or literature. You must contact individual universities for their specific entry requirements. See www.britishcouncil.org or www.ielts.org for information on IELTS, preparation for the test, test centres and how to apply to take the test.

Overseas-trained nurse or midwife from within the EU/EEA

If you are a registered nurse and trained within the EU/EEA, you can consult the 'Joining the register' section of the NMC website (www.nmc-uk.org/Registration/Joining-the-register) for details of how to gain the NMC registration needed to practise as a nurse or midwife in the UK. There is a £110 fee to have an application assessed and the process can take three to six months.

You can check on the NMC website to see whether your qualification is one that leads to automatic recognition. If not, you will be required to send transcripts of your course, so that the NMC can compare it against UK educational requirements.

You may be required to undertake a period of adaptation, or sit an aptitude test. Adaptation can involve doing an approved EU Nurse Adaptation programme. The NMC website approved programmes database (www.nmc-uk.org/Approved-Programmes) will help you locate EU Nurse Adaptation programmes.

Overseas-trained nurse or midwife from outside the EU/EEA

If you trained outside the EU/EEA, including in the USA, you need to be a registered nurse or midwife and have at least 12 months' registered practice in the field of nursing to which you want to apply. The application-for-assessment fee is £140. You must also have a minimum score of

7.0 on IELTS. This is a strict requirement irrespective of whether you are a British citizen or your first language is English.

The course you studied overseas would also have to match NMC requirements in terms of length and number of practice hours. If your course meets the criteria, you would then have to do an Overseas Nursing programme. Use the NMC website approved programmes database to locate Overseas Nursing programmes and the single Overseas Midwives programme on offer.

Check carefully, as some programmes offered by universities for overseas nurses may have lower English-language requirements but fail to lead to NMC registration; such programmes may be more suitable if you want to return to nursing in the country where you trained.

What if I want to top up my diploma in nursing to a degree?

From September 2013 the entry route for new nurses will be by degree only and registered nurses who qualified through on a diploma course may wish to top up their qualifications to a degree, perhaps for career progression. Currently, Buckinghamshire New University, the University of Sunderland, the University of West London and the University of Dundee offer one-year top-up or conversion courses for registered nurses with post-qualifying experience, who either trained through the diploma route or through an earlier qualification. It is also possible to study parts of these courses as stand-alone modules as part of continuing professional development (CPD). There are both taught and work-based modules. Other universities may consider taking diploma-qualified students onto the second year of a nursing degree.

You can use UCAS to locate one-year top-up courses. Private-education providers, such as BPP University College, may also offer top-up degrees.

What if I wish to return to nursing after a break?

If you were previously registered as a nurse or midwife in the UK but have had a break from working, you should contact the NMC to see what you would need to do to rejoin the register. You may need to complete a number of practice hours or complete a return-to-practice programme. Use the NMC website approved programmes database to search for Return to Practice courses.

Studying nursing or midwifery abroad

Although it is possible to study for a nursing or midwifery degree out-side the UK, if you then want to return to practise in the UK, you must be aware of the requirements of the NMC registration process.

If you study within the EU/EEA, you will need to have studied a course approved by the NMC that leads to automatic recognition. You can use the NMC website to identify courses that lead to automatic recognition. If your course doesn't qualify, you may have to spend time and money doing an adaptation course or sit an aptitude test before you can regis-ter to practise as a nurse or midwife in the UK.

The following websites may be useful to find nursing and midwifery courses in the EU: www.eunicas.co.uk and www.astarfuture.co.uk. There are no fees for UK students who wish to study in the four Scandinavian countries, and fees can be lower in other parts of the EU than in the UK. However, you must bear in mind that you would not benefit from an NHS bursary and although courses are often taught in English, on placement you would have to converse with patients in their native language.

If you choose to study outside the EU/EEA, including in the USA, you would need 12 months' registered practice as a nurse or midwife, be able to meet English-language requirements (irrespective of whether English is your first language) and also have to do an Overseas Nursing programme before you could register to practise in the UK. See the NMC website, www.nmc-uk.org, for full details.

If you want to spend some time studying abroad, it may be better to consider a nursing or midwifery degree that offers an elective place-ment abroad. Universities often have partnership agreements with uni-versities overseas, such as through the Erasmus scheme, www.britishcouncil.org/erasmus.htm, or they can help arrange placements to allow students to volunteer abroad or to experience healthcare in other countries.

9 | Results day

Results for A levels are published in the third week in August and are available to collect from schools and colleges on the third Thursday in August. Scottish Higher results come out in early August; check the Scottish Qualifications Authority (SQA) website (www.sqa.org.uk) for the exact date.

> **TIP**
>
> Make sure that you are available on results day; you may need to speak to universities to make quick and important decisions about your future. Universities may insist on speaking to you, not to your parents.

It is better to collect the results yourself, rather than wait for your school or college to post the results slip to you, so that you can act quickly if you haven't quite made the grades and need to contact universities or make any important decisions. This chapter contains the information that you need in order to be prepared when your results arrive so that you know what to do (depending on your situation) and it will take you through the steps you should follow if you don't do as well as expected.

How to be prepared

Before results day it is important to check that:

* UCAS have your correct contact details, especially if there have been any changes
* you have your UCAS login details – so that you will be able to check on UCAS Track whether you have been accepted
* you have the telephone numbers for both your firm-offer and insurance-offer universities; if you cannot get through on these numbers, you may have to use a central Clearing number which universities will display on their websites and on UCAS Clearing information; it is important to have all these contact details to hand, to ensure that you have the best chance to get through to a university if necessary.

How do universities get my results?

UCAS will receive your results and send them to universities; this includes A levels, Scottish Highers and Advanced Highers. For some qualifications you will have to send your results yourself direct to individual universities. If in doubt, the UCAS website has a list of qualifications they automatically send to universities on your behalf at www. ucas.com/students/results/examresults.

Universities receive some results before applicants so by the time you have your results, they may have made a decision regarding whether to make you an offer. Universities then notify UCAS of their decisions, and the decisions are displayed on UCAS Track. See the UCAS website for useful information on the messages you can expect to appear on your Track account on results day and on what to do.

Typical situations and what to do

The following are situations you may find yourself in on results day and what you should do.

I've got the grades for my firm choice

If you meet all of the conditions of your firm offer, you will be accepted by your firm-choice university. It may take some time for this to be confirmed on Track but you do not need to do anything! You can relax and wait for a congratulations message on Track and a confirmation letter from UCAS. The university will then contact you with accommodation and registration details.

I've missed my firm choice by one grade

If you have not quite met the requirements of your offer, for example, missing by one A level grade, you may find that the university has still accepted you. If, however, you haven't had your place confirmed on Track, you should get on the phone to your firm-choice university to see whether they may still consider you. In some cases, universities will allow applicants who hold a conditional offer to slip a grade (particularly if they came across well at the interview stage) rather than offer the place to somebody else. It may be difficult to get through to the university but if they can see you are still keen and you can perhaps explain why you didn't quite achieve the grades you hoped for, they may still offer you a place. Ringing universities at this time can be stressful but it is important that you do this, perhaps with help from a teacher or careers adviser.

When you speak to the universities, they are likely to give you a simple 'yes' or 'no' answer, or tell you that you are still being considered. If they tell you that you have been rejected, ask how they would view an application from you in the following year. If they then give you a positive response about reapplying, seek to get it confirmed in writing, as this will give you hard evidence of their intention to consider your application again.

I've got the grades for my insurance choice

If you didn't get the grades for your first choice but did for your insurance choice, you will be accepted there and just need to wait for confirmation on UCAS Track.

I didn't meet the grades for either of my offers

If you did not meet the conditions of either your firm or insurance choice, you automatically go into Clearing (see page 100).

I've got better grades than expected

If you do better than expected and get higher grades than needed for your firm choice, you may be eligible for Adjustment. UCAS says that you are eligible if you have met and exceeded your original conditional firm-offer conditions. Adjustment is available from A level results day to 31 August. An option will appear on UCAS Track to register for Adjustment. This is only possible for your firm choice. It means that you have a short period of time, around five days, to look for vacancies and trade up for another course.

If you are happy with the place you have already secured, there is no need to do anything. Bear in mind that it is highly unlikely that you will be successful in finding vacancies on nursing and midwifery courses at this time of year as most courses will be full. If, however, you have decided that you no longer want to study nursing or midwifery, alternative courses may be available through Adjustment.

I've been made a changed-course offer

If you weren't successful in getting a place on a nursing or midwifery course, you may be offered an alternative course at the same university. You are not obliged to accept this. You must think carefully before you reply and seek help from your school or college or from a careers adviser. Bear in mind that you may have the option to reapply for nursing or midwifery in the following year.

I've changed my mind about my firm choice

If you change your mind and no longer want to go to your firm choice and would prefer to go to your insurance choice, you must be aware that in accepting a firm offer in the first place you made a commitment to going there. You will need to contact your firm-choice university as soon as possible to see whether they will withdraw your offer, although it may take some time to get through to them by phone. You should then contact your insurance choice to see whether they are still able to take you through Clearing; this is not certain as they will no longer be holding a place for you even if you had met the conditions of your offer. By this time your place may have been offered to someone else and they may not have any other vacancies.

You should think carefully about these decisions and seek help from your school, college or a careers adviser. Don't accept a place at a university where you feel you will be unhappy but equally be aware that if you don't accept this place, you can't guarantee that other places will still be available to you. There are some very useful FAQs on the UCAS website (www.ucas.com/students/offers/faqs) to help with this.

I don't hold any offers

There are a number of students who will approach results day without having received an offer from a nursing or midwifery course. In the past, if you found yourself in this position and secured good grades in your A levels, it may have been possible to find a place through Clearing. Unfortunately, it is now virtually impossible to secure a place on a course in this way, even if you have outstanding grades. This is because nursing and midwifery courses are so popular and universities have often filled their places early on in the year. This situation is unlikely to change in the coming years. Ultimately, though, Clearing may be of use to secure a place on an alternative course if you decide that you no longer want to study nursing or midwifery. If this is the case, you should speak to a careers adviser or members of staff at your school or college before you make any decisions.

Clearing

If you are eligible for Clearing, an 'Add Clearing Choice' button will appear on UCAS Track with your personal Clearing number; UCAS no longer sends confirmation of eligibility for Clearing in the post. You need to look at course vacancies, published in *The Telegraph* and on the UCAS website, and then contact universities that interest you. Make sure that you have your Clearing number to hand; this will allow universities to view your application. Don't feel that you have to accept the first informal offer you are given over the phone. When you have decided which offer to accept, enter these details on Track. When the university accepts you, confirmation of this will appear on Track.

Remarks and appeals

If you are considering having any of your exams remarked, you should first seek some advice from your school or college. Applicants who use the remark and appeal services have no guarantee that universities will wait for the remark or appeal and keep their offers of places on courses open.

Retaking A levels

You need to seek advice from your school or college about retake costs and timings or whether you need to study for an additional year. Your tutors will be able to advise whether in an extra year you will realistically achieve the grades you need or whether you should revise your choice of universities or courses.

You should also contact individual universities to see whether their grade requirements are likely to be higher than when you originally applied and whether they accept applications with retake grades.

Reapplying

If you have been unsuccessful in getting a place, the main option you have is to reapply through UCAS in the next admissions cycle. Although you will already have the grades for entry in this situation, you must bear in mind that grade requirements can change each year and that there are a number of other elements of your application that you'll need to work on to maximise your chances of securing a place. You need to consider the following elements.

- Your personal statement – revisit it and cast a critical eye over it. This is also an opportunity to add in any work placements or other positive experiences that you have had since you made your application.
- Your work experience – any opportunity to add further work experience to your profile will always be a good step. Whether it is health-related or just general voluntary work, it will have a positive impact.
- Review the feedback you got from any failed interviews.

The only safe method of finding out whether a university will consider a reapplication is to call or email to ask. It is often worth doing this by email so that you have firm details of what has been discussed to refer back to at a later time if necessary. Make sure that you find out the appropriate person to send this to, probably the admissions tutor for the course. The format of your email should be:

- your previous UCAS number
- opening paragraph to explain your circumstances – for example, applied last year and given an offer but didn't meet the grades/ rejected after interview/rejected without an interview
- your exam results and what you hope to improve on (if appropriate)
- any circumstances which affected your performance in exams (if appropriate, you may also wish to include a letter or statement from your school to back this up)
- your retake plan – including the timescale, also any additional work experience you hope to undertake
- a request for advice as to whether you would be considered.

10 | Fees and funding

There has been discussion in the news recently about a greater number of universities deciding to charge maximum tuition fees. The good news is that UK students accepted onto a full-time or part-time course that leads to professional registration as a nurse or midwife (both undergraduate and postgraduate routes) are eligible for an NHS bursary package which includes payment of your tuition fees by the NHS.

However, there are other costs associated with going to university; so in this chapter we will look at a breakdown of the financial help you can expect to receive; how it compares in England, Wales, Scotland and Northern Ireland; and how to apply. We will look at sponsorship opportunities for healthcare assistants wishing to train as a nurse, and for becoming a nurse or midwife in the armed forces. Finally, there is some information on alternative sources of funding for which you may be eligible to apply.

NHS bursaries

NHS bursaries are available to UK students accepted onto a full-time or part-time course that leads to professional registration as a nurse or midwife (both undergraduate and postgraduate routes). The bursary package includes payment of tuition fees by the NHS, an income-assessed NHS bursary and additional allowances for eligible students. In addition, in England and Wales you can also apply for a non-income-assessed student loan, to help with living costs. Help provided is broadly comparable in England, Wales, Scotland and Northern Ireland but is administered by different organisations. See later in this chapter for more details.

You must bear in mind that NHS bursaries are not available for post-registration courses.

Applicants for NHS bursaries also need to satisfy residency requirements. EU nationals who have not been ordinarily resident in the UK are eligible to have only their fees paid, and students from outside the EEA are not eligible for any part of the NHS bursary.

How to apply for an NHS bursary

For students studying nursing or midwifery in England

When you have been made an offer by a university, either conditional or unconditional, the university will advise NHS Student Bursaries who will contact you with information on how to apply for a bursary using the Bursary Online Support System (BOSS). This involves paying a fee and sending supporting documentation.

Currently the NHS bursary means that:

* your course fees are paid
* you receive a £1,000 non-income-assessed grant.

If you are living away from your parental home:

* you receive an income-assessed basic bursary of £2,591 (30-week course) plus £82 for each additional week of your course (maximum payable £4,395).

If you are living in your parental home:

* you receive an income-assessed basic bursary of £2,163 (30-week course) plus £54 for each additional week of your course (maximum payable £3,351).

If you are living in London (either in or away from your parental home):

* you receive an income-assessed basic bursary of £3,128 (30-week course) plus £106 for each additional week of your course (maximum payable £5,460).

Check the NHS Student Bursaries website (www.nhsbsa.nhs.uk/Students) for figures on how your parents', spouse's or partner's income will affect the amount you receive. Remember, even if you don't think you will be eligible for an income-assessed bursary, you must apply to NHS Student Bursaries to have your fees paid and to receive the non-income-assessed grant.

If you are eligible, you can also claim:

* dependants allowance
* parent learning allowance
* childcare allowance
* disabled student allowance.

See www.nhsbsa.nhs.uk/Students for more details and eligibility criteria.

You may also get assistance with placement costs, including travel and possibly accommodation. You should contact the university to which you are applying for advice on how to claim.

Please bear in mind that these are the current figures and may change annually. Full details and eligibility criteria can be found on the NHS Student Bursaries website, where you can also download the booklet *Financial Help for Healthcare Students*. You can use a student-bursary calculator on this website to work out what you could receive.

For students studying nursing or midwifery in Wales

For students in Wales the NHS bursary means that:

- your course fees are paid
- you receive a non-means-tested grant of £1,000.

If you are living away from your parental home:

- you receive a means-tested basic bursary of £2,591 (30-week course) plus £82 for each additional week of your course (maximum payable £4,395).

If you are living in your parental home:

- you receive a means-tested basic bursary of £2,163 (30-week course) plus £54 for each additional week of your course (maximum payable £3,351).

See NHS Wales Student Award Unit (www.wales.nhs.uk/sitesplus/829/page/36092) for more details of how much your means-tested bursary will be reduced based on your parents', spouse's or partner's income.

If you are eligible, you can also claim:

- dependants allowance
- parent learning allowance
- childcare allowance
- disabled student allowance.

See NHS Wales Student Award Unit for more details and eligibility criteria.

You may also get assistance with placement costs, which are income-assessed. You should contact the university to which you are applying for advice on how to claim.

For further information, see the NHS Wales Student Award Unit. Please bear in mind that these are the current rates and may change annually. If you are offered a university place, the NHS Wales Student Award Unit will contact you with application details.

For students studying nursing or midwifery in Scotland

The Nursing and Midwifery Students Bursary Scheme (NMSB) means that:

- your course fees are paid
- you receive a full bursary of £6,578 for Years 1–3 of your course, with £4,938 for Year 4; there is also a £60 initial-expenses allowance in Year 1.

If you are eligible, you can also claim:

- dependants allowance
- single parent allowance

- childcare allowance
- disabled student allowance.

See the Student Award Agency for Scotland (SAAS) at www.saas.gov.uk for more details and eligibility criteria.

Expenses for placements may also be payable. Ask for a form to claim from the university where you are going to study or download one from SAAS.

Please bear in mind that these are the current figures and may change annually. Contact SAAS for further details of the NMSB. Apply online to SAAS as soon as you get a letter of acceptance of a place from a university. If you are not a UK or EU national, you must have settled-residency status in the UK on the relevant date to be eligible for this bursary scheme.

For students studying nursing or midwifery in Northern Ireland

A Health and Social Care (HSC) bursary may be available for UK or European Community/EEA nationals. Contact Nursing and Midwifery Careers in Northern Ireland (www.nursingandmidwiferycareersni.com) for the current rate.

Student loan

English students

If you normally live in England, regardless of where in the UK you are going to study, you may be eligible for a reduced-rate, non-means-tested student loan from Student Finance England, www.studentfinanceengland.co.uk. The NHS bursary is not intended to meet all your requirements, so you are encouraged to consider carefully whether you need this additional loan.

A new NHS student starting a course from 1 September 2013 can get up to a £3,263 maintenance loan from Student Finance England. This needs to be paid back when you are earning over £21,000 per year. Apply at www.sfengland.slc.co.uk.

Welsh students

If you normally live in Wales, regardless of where in the UK you are going to study, you may be eligible for a reduced-rate, non-means-tested maintenance loan.

If you are living away from your parental home:

- you receive a non-means-tested maintenance loan of £2,324.

If you are living in your parental home:

- you receive a non-means-tested maintenance loan of £1,744.

Contact your local authority for information on the amount of your possible entitlement. Applications can be made through Student Finance Wales (www.studentfinancewales.co.uk).

How to apply for a student loan

As soon as you have applied to UCAS, you can make a start on your application for a student loan, which needs to be completed by 31 May to make sure that you have your loan when you start the course in autumn.

Scottish students

Students who receive support from the Nursing and Midwifery Students Bursary Scheme (NMSB) are not eligible for a student loan.

Northern Ireland students

Students who receive a Health and Social Care (HSC) bursary are not eligible for a student loan.

EU students

EU students who satisfy residency criteria and have settled status in the UK may be eligible for an NHS bursary. EU students who do not have a right of permanent residence in the UK may be eligible to have their tuition fees paid but not receive the NHS bursary maintenance loan. EU students are not normally eligible for student loans. See Financial Help for Health Care Students, downloadable from the NHS Student Bursaries website (www.nhsbsa.nhs.uk/Students), for more details.

International students

Students from outside the EEA are not eligible for any part of the NHS bursary. For this reason, in almost all cases, they are not eligible to apply for pre-registration nursing and midwifery courses. See the section on international students in Chapter 8. If places are available, students from outside the EEA would need to pay international student fees, so they should to contact individual universities for details.

Sponsorship opportunities

It can sometimes be possible to have a pre-registration nursing or midwifery course funded by an employer as part of an employment contract or for career progression.

Healthcare assistants

The NHS can sometimes offer secondments to healthcare assistants or assistant practitioners (more experienced healthcare assistants) to train as a nurse. A seconded student will normally receive basic pay from the NHS but would not be eligible for a bursary, and may be expected to work for the NHS Trust that has seconded them for a set period after completing their course. See the NHS Careers website (www.nhscareers.nhs.uk) for more details.

Armed-forces nurses

If you want to work in the army, the Queen Alexandra's Royal Army Nursing Corps (QARANC) recruits and then sponsors students to study a BSc in Adult or Mental Health Nursing at Birmingham City University. Initial basic military training precedes studying to be a nurse. You are employed by the army and paid a wage whilst at university. Entry is competitive, see www.army.mod.uk for more details and check with Birmingham City University for entry requirements; currently you need the equivalent of 280 UCAS points for the nursing degree.

You can become a Medical Naval Nurse, through the Queen Alexandra's Royal Naval Nursing Service (QARNNS). You spend 10 weeks on basic navy training and then are sponsored to complete a BSc in Nursing at Birmingham City University. See royalnavy.mod.uk/careers for more details.

Similarly, you can join the Princess Mary's Royal Air Force Nursing Service (PMRAFNS) to be sponsored on a BSc in Nursing at Birmingham City University. Placements include both NHS and military establishments. See www.raf.mod.uk/careers for more details.

Other sources of financial help

The National Scholarship Programme

This scholarship programme is for students whose family income is less than £25,000 per year and wish to study at a university in England. The universities decide who is to receive this award. Use the UCAS website course search to see information on individual universities or contact universities for details.

Access to Learning Funds

If you have taken up your entitlement to a bursary and student loan and you need further financial support, you can apply to the Access to Learning Fund at the university where you have chosen to study. Ask for

further details from the universities you are applying to or visit www.gov.
uk/access-to-learning-fund/overview.

Council tax

Full-time students are usually exempt from council tax or are entitled to
discounts; see www.gov.uk/council-tax/full-time-students. In excep-
tional circumstances, you may be eligible for housing benefit and other
benefits.

Scholarships

Contact individual universities for details of possible scholarships or
bursaries for which you may be able to apply. Bursary and scholarship
information can be found by using the UCAS website course search
(www.ucas.com) to find information on individual universities. You can
also use www.scholarship-search.org.uk. Here are just two examples.

* The University of York offers a York Annual Fund Bursary, for
  students from low family-income backgrounds. This is a £1,000
  single payment.
* The University of West London offers academic merit awards of up
  to £1,000 for nursing and midwifery students.

See the Royal College of Nursing website (www.rcn.org.uk) for details
of RCN Foundation Bursaries. These include the Margaret Parkinson
Scholarship. This is an annual award to encourage graduates with a
non-nursing degree to qualify as a registered nurse by studying a degree
in nursing. An award of £500–£2,000 is made to an individual each year
for up to three years. This should not affect the amount you receive in
your NHS bursary.

Educational Grants Search

Educational grants are aimed at individuals on low incomes or those
from low-income families to enable them to start a course or to support
existing students to complete their studies. Small grants of between
£200 and £500 can sometimes be awarded to those who are eligible.
See www.family-action.org.uk.

Cavell Nurses Trust

The Cavell Nurses Trust supports student nurses who need financial
help following illness, injury and other difficulties. There are also five
categories of scholarship awards for which second-year or third-year
nurses can apply. See www.cavellnursestrust.org for more information.

> **TIP**
>
> Be aware that if you are sponsored or in receipt of a scholarship, bursary or an amount other than a Student Loan or Access to Learning Funds payment, you will not be eligible for an NHS bursary if your income exceeds the maximum bursary amount. See www.nhsbsa.nhs.uk for more details.

11| Careers

This chapter begins with the first step to be taken after you have graduated, namely, registration with the NMC, and then provides a brief overview of current employment prospects for nurses and midwives.

The aim of the main section of the chapter is to help you further confirm which branch of nursing you should choose or whether midwifery is right for you. We will look at each area of nursing in detail, what the job can involve, settings you can work in and the specialist roles you could perform. Case studies from current nursing students and a newly qualified nurse will give you a further insight into what each type of nursing can be like. We will similarly look at what midwives do, where they can work and the specialist roles they can move into, including a case study of a newly qualified midwife.

The chapter continues with details of a wide range of career routes for newly qualified or experienced nurses and the branch of nursing or type of experience which is most suitable for each.

The chapter concludes with progression routes into management; teaching and assessing; research; and consultant-level posts for both nurses and midwives. Professional development and opportunities for further study will be covered as well as the levels of salary you can expect. There are also sections on working overseas and opportunities in the armed forces.

Once you have graduated: NMC registration

After completing your course, you will need to register with the NMC before you can practise as a nurse or midwife. On receiving notification from a university that a student has completed an approved nursing or midwifery course, the NMC sends a registration application pack to the applicant to be returned to them with a £100 fee. See www.nmc-uk.org for more information on registration.

Employment prospects

Nurses make up the largest group of professionals in the NHS. According to the NHS Information Centre, in September 2012 there were around 314,377 qualified nurses working in the NHS. There were also 26,225 midwives, 10,361 health visitors and 1,519 school nurses (NHS Hospital and Community Health Service monthly workforce statistics September 2012).

Cuts to healthcare spending have meant a reduction in the number of nursing posts in some areas of the country and overall in the last year the number of qualified nurses working in the sector has fallen by around 0.6%. However, in many cases Healthcare Trusts have sought to minimise the effects on front-line jobs such as nursing and midwifery and have instead cut administrative and managerial roles or made savings in other ways. There has been an increase in the number of posts for midwives, health visitors and school nurses. Currently there is a drive to recruit more health visitors.

For many years, public perception has regarded the NHS to be the traditional employer of nurses and midwives. Whilst this is certainly a big part of the employment picture, it is certainly not the whole picture. Nurses, in particular, are increasingly working in the community. There are moves to provide more care outside hospitals in the community, 24-hour care and more services for the elderly, who are a growing part of the population. According to the Royal College of Nursing, around one third of their members work in the independent sector. A substantial number of nurses and midwives work in the armed forces.

Finding a job

During your course you should begin to consider where you would like to work when you qualify. Keep a record of the placements you have completed and how you felt about particular areas of nursing or midwifery and different settings. Keep any details of useful contacts for when you start searching for jobs. There are no hard and fast rules on which areas of nursing or midwifery you should choose to begin your career, but certain posts may require applicants to have post-registration experience and some settings may be more suitable for a first post. For example, settings where you would be working in a team rather than as an autonomous professional may be an easier transition from training, such as a midwife choosing to work in a hospital rather than in the community.

You will need to search for possible vacancies. Useful sources of job vacancies are:

- www.jobs.nhs.uk
- www.nursingtimesjobs.com
- www.rcnbulletinjobs.co.uk
- http://jobs.midwives.co.uk
- www.staffnurse.com
- www.nursing-personnel.co.uk.

If you have qualified and do not yet have a job, you can use the NHS Jobs Service for newly qualified healthcare professionals: www.jobs. nhs.uk/news/latest12.html. You log onto NHS jobs and register your details with your local Newly Qualified Profile Pool; you will then be sent NHS job opportunities.

First year as a nurse or midwife

Once you have completed your course and registered with the NMC, you will typically follow this career path during your first year.

Preceptorship

Nurses and midwives in the NHS begin their first post with a period of preceptorship, similar to a probationary period, which usually lasts around 6 to 12 months. During this time new members of staff receive supervision and support to ease them into their new roles and to ensure that they are competent practitioners. They will be supervised by a preceptor, a qualified and suitably experienced practitioner. All new staff should have the opportunity to reach specific competencies that relate to their specific role as well as development opportunities in leadership, management and working in multidisciplinary teams.

Preceptorships differ according to each NHS Trust but usually include regular meetings with a preceptor and opportunities for learning, such as dedicated study days. Newly qualified staff should expect development reviews at 6 and 12 months and at each of these points, if they have reached a satisfactory level of practice, should move up a pay point. Flying Start England is a national development programme for all newly qualified nurses and midwives and acts as a useful online resource during a preceptorship. See www.flyingstartengland.nhs.uk for more details.

The majority of newly qualified nurses or midwives start their careers working in the NHS but it may also be possible to work in the independent sector, such as for a private healthcare provider or a charity. Outside the NHS there is no obligation for employers to provide a preceptorship, although the Royal College of Nursing and the Royal College of Midwives recommend that employers should.

Maintaining your NMC registration

To maintain registration with the NMC, nurses and midwives need to meet post-registration education and practice (PREP) standards. The standards are there to 'safeguard the health and wellbeing of the public by ensuring that anyone renewing their registration has undertaken a minimum amount of practice'. In order to maintain their NMC registration, nurses and midwives are expected to have practised for a minimum of 450 hours during the three years prior to the renewal of their registration. They will also need to have completed 35 hours of learning activity as continuing professional development (CPD) during the three years prior to renewal of registration. They must also keep a personal professional profile or portfolio of the learning activities in which they have been involved.

Salaries

Most nurses and midwives begin their careers by working in the NHS. As one of the largest employers in the UK, the NHS has clearly defined pay bands for nurses and midwives. The Agenda for Change pay system sets out the salary grades for posts and these are matched to the abilities and responsibilities a nurse or midwife has developed in their work role. New nurses and midwives enter their professions at Level 5 in the NHS and may progress beyond the starting point of this entry band once they have had their first appraisal.

The following are examples of Agenda for Change pay rates from 1 April 2013:

- nurse: Band 5 (£21,388–£27,901)
- midwife: starting point Band 5 (£21,388), can rise to Band 6 (£25,783–£34,530)
- nurse specialist or nurse team leader: Band 6 (£25,738–£34,530)
- health visitor: Band 6 (£25,738–£34,530)
- nurse advanced or midwife higher level/research projects or midwife team manager: Band 7 (£30,764–£40,588)
- modern matron: Band 8a (£39,239–£47,088)
- nurse or midwife consultant: Band 8a–c (can earn up to £67,805).

High cost area supplements are available for those working in and around London.

Current NHS pay bands can be viewed at www.nhscareers.nhs.uk/working-in-the-nhs/pay-and-benefits/agenda-for-change-pay-rates.

Pay is comparable in private healthcare. You may find www.privatehealth.co.uk/jobs and www.privatehealthcareers.co.uk useful sources of information.

Career choices for nurses and midwives

The following information may give you further help in choosing to study a branch of nursing or deciding to study midwifery. We will look at the specialist areas or job roles that are possible in each branch of nursing and in midwifery, and progression routes that are open to all nurses and midwives.

Adult nursing

What do adult nurses do?

Adult nurses work with a wide range of people, from young adults to the elderly, with both long-term and short-term health conditions. Adult nursing is sometimes called general nursing and has some overlaps with other branches of nursing. It can include working with babies; children and young people; pregnant and post-natal women; those with mental-health problems; those with physical disabilities; and people with long-term problems such as cognitive impairment. You need to be interested in learning how to treat lots of different conditions and in learning practical clinical skills. You also need to enjoy working with adults and their families. It can be busy, fast changing and demanding and it requires good teamworking.

The care that adult nurses give includes:

- making accurate assessments of individual patient needs and writing, implementing and evaluating care plans
- being alert to early signs of illness in people of all ages
- helping patients meet their personal needs, such as washing and toileting, making sure that patients are comfortable in stressful situations
- monitoring temperature, pulse, blood pressure, oxygen levels, respiration rate, making physical examinations and treating wounds
- ensuring that patients have adequate nutritional and fluid intake
- administering medicines and sometimes prescribing medicines, explaining benefits and risks
- administering injections, taking blood, inserting an IV cannula to administer fluids through a vein
- basic or advanced resuscitation
- using complex life-support equipment
- palliative care
- promoting self-care, particularly for people with long-term conditions
- teaching or educating patients, families and others
- leading, coordinating, delegating and supervising care
- shared decision making with other professional healthcare workers.

Adult nurses have a key role in promoting good health and well-being through education. As with other areas of nursing practice, adult nurses plan and deliver care within a multidisciplinary team; they are frequently the main point of contact with patients.

An important point to consider when thinking about becoming an adult nurse is that the people they support are usually unwell. Some areas of nursing or healthcare focus on psychological or social aspects of health – these are very important – but for adult nurses, much time is spent in supporting people who are physically ill. There are specialist nurses for a huge number of conditions, such as diabetes and motor neurone disease, and within specialist departments, such as oncology (cancer care) and cardiology (disorders of the heart), and within new areas such as tuberculosis (TB).

Case study

Holly Southall completed an adult nursing degree at De Montfort University and is in her first job at Leicester Royal Hospital.

I chose adult nursing because it is a very broad area to work in with opportunities to specialise in areas such as diabetes, cardiology and care of the elderly to name but a few. Because it's so broad it's inevitable that you will gain experience which can be applied elsewhere and it is easy to progress to a wide range of different jobs and settings as training is readily offered.

I work as a staff nurse in the surgical intensive care unit (ITU) at Leicester Royal which feeds from the Royal's Accident and Emergency Department (A&E), one of the busiest A&Es in Europe. I look after people who are critically ill due to an unexpected incident, so a broad knowledge is needed. This can include people who have been in RTAs (road traffic accidents), had an emergency operation, have sepsis (blood infection), binge drinkers, attempted suicides and people who have taken overdoses, victims of assaults and women who have complications during labour.

Usually patients have one or more failing organ systems within their body. Most of our patients are ventilated and sedated, so we can take over their breathing, some also have support to maintain their blood pressure and a type of filtration used to remove waste products from their blood if their kidneys begin to fail. The role is one of contrasts; we have to understand and use high-tech machines but on the other hand carry out basic nursing care such as washing a patient, moving a patient's body to prevent pressure sores and mouth care, such as cleaning teeth and dentures as our patients are so ill they cannot perform any of these tasks for themselves. An important part of the role is supporting a patient's relatives at what is a traumatic time for families.

Nobody can prepare a person sufficiently for the first time they see their family member on a life-support machine. An ITU nurse has to be there sometimes for a shoulder to cry on or sometimes to be shouted at by families.

The most enjoyable thing about the job is that every day is different, patients' outcomes may not always be positive but there is the satisfaction in having done the best you can for that patient and their family.

Adult nurses within the healthcare system

We think of adult nurses as primarily working in hospitals and although there will always be hospital roles that involve working with specific patient groups, there are important factors that are driving changes relevant to adult nursing.

- Hospital care is very expensive.
- Treatments are increasingly successful: people are now much more likely to survive serious illness or trauma. This, combined with the general rise in life expectancy, means that the health needs of the ageing population are escalating and will continue to do so.
- Hospital care is aimed at people who are very ill and are not always able to fight infections. Where possible, avoiding hospital helps decrease further acquisition of infection.
- For many people, especially the old and frail, being in hospital disrupts routine. Unfamiliar surroundings often increase confusion, and distance from home means that family or friends cannot easily offer personal support.

Because of these and many other factors, there is now a steady shift in the emphasis of care towards the community, with people who would previously have been occupying a general-hospital bed now being cared for in their own homes. Many of these people have at least one long-term condition, or health disruptions which are often lifelong and limit the quality of life; such conditions mostly cannot be cured but can be controlled. However, those affected often experience severe limitations on their lifestyles – they have difficulty with personal care, mobility and daily activities, such as getting dressed, housework or preparing a meal.

A key adult-nursing role is to support patients remaining in their own home rather than being admitted to hospital; this is achieved by assessing need, planning care, providing support and facilitating care by other agencies, such as social-service teams or voluntary organisations contracted to provide home-care services. Adult nurses can be found in primary-care settings, such as GP surgeries and health centres as well as in community-care settings, such as nursing homes and working for charities.

Specialist roles for adult nurses

Intensive care

In intensive care, patients are supported by complex life-support and monitoring equipment to (often artificially) maintain respiration, cardiac function and renal function. Patients are cared for by experienced adult nurses on a one-to-one basis, 24 hours a day. In addition to being able to use technical equipment and administer complex medication, nurses in this area must also ensure high standards of personal patient care, liaise with patients' families in difficult circumstances and work closely with many other health professionals. Decisions about care often need to be made very quickly and intuition is a key skill.

Accident and Emergency (A&E)

Some adult nurses specialise in working in Accident and Emergency Departments (A&E) and emergency-admissions wards. The pace of activity in A&E can vary dramatically, and you can be dealing with anything from routine cuts and sprains to major burns and cardiac arrest. The nursing care required is inevitably varied and change can be unpredictable – you need to think quickly. In addition to managing the care needed, nurses also have responsibilities for the related needs of patient and family, including anxiety, fear, loss and grieving.

Other areas of hospitals that adult nurses may work in are:

- theatre and surgical wards
- neonatal care
- with patients with acute conditions – such as heart failure, stroke, hepatitis, burns
- neurology
- women's or men's health
- cancer care
- respiratory care.

Nursing homes

Care is led and managed by nurses who use their professional judgement to enable people to regain, improve or maintain health or to achieve the best possible quality at the end of their life. Nurses work closely with patients and their families and other health staff. A key role for adult nurses is to continually assess the needs of patients, then to make detailed plans of care, much of which will be delivered by other care staff that the adult nurse will supervise. Additionally, there is complex medication to administer, dressings and other treatments to give whilst at all times being aware of the need to safeguard the vulnerable people in their care.

Treating patients with chronic conditions

This can involve assessing patients in their own homes or in a clinic and then helping to coordinate care and specialist rehabilitation services in order to address symptoms. Adult nurses in this area support patients, families and carers. Adult nurses who support people with a long-term condition (such as diabetes and heart/kidney problems) work inter-professionally to enable patients to remain at home and live independently as long as possible. They provide one-to-one education to help patients manage their own care and medication.

Children's nursing

What do children's nurses do?

Children's nurses deliver professional nursing care to children from birth to adolescence. They seek to improve a child's health for life, to reduce the likelihood of illness and hospitalisation. You would need to enjoy both being and playing with children but equally supporting and educating parents and carers. You need to have a good understanding of child development. It is also important to be alert and observant; when children are sick, particularly babies, they can deteriorate rapidly.

A key factor in successfully nursing children and supporting their families is communication. Most adults, even if they are unwell, are able to describe how they are feeling physically, for example, describing pain, and are able to express their concerns, for example, their mood or their fear of dying. Younger children, especially, cannot easily articulate what they feel. The skills learnt in children's-nurse training include strategies and techniques to identify, assess and interpret a child's behaviours and make rapid decisions based on the evidence the nurse sees. You need to be intuitive and good at interpreting non-verbal communication.

Nursing a child is diverse, and children have not just physical-health needs but also emotional, learning and developmental needs. You may have to deal with distressed children or parents, and the job can be emotionally demanding. The role involves working in partnership with many other health professionals, parents, families and carers.

The role may involve:

- working in partnership with the child, parents and carers, supporting parents with having a child in hospital and managing care for the child when they return home
- clinical procedures, recording pulse, temperature and respiration, wound care, setting up drips and giving blood transfusions
- using play or distraction techniques
- understanding legalities of parental consent and being able to explain these clearly

- acting as an advocate for children to support their rights to be safe and to reach their full potential
- working with children with physical disabilities or learning disabilities
- promoting physical, emotional and sexual health
- making accurate medicines' dosage calculations
- safeguarding children
- preparing children for operations and procedures, where they may be very frightened.

Case study

Victoria Lynne is a third-year children's nursing student at Birmingham City University. Her experiences on placement may help you better understand the role of a children's nurse.

I chose children's nursing because I wanted to help children and families at some of the most vulnerable times in their lives. I was attracted to working with a wide age range; the role can involve working with babies to young adults at different stages of development, with needs and conditions that all bring their own challenges.

The biggest challenge I have faced on placement so far has been reacting to an emergency situation in the high dependency area of a neonatal surgical ward. I was on a night shift when a baby that was a few hours' old was transferred to the ward from the district general hospital, with gastroschisis (born with his intestines outside of his body). He was being monitored by a machine to measure oxygen-saturation levels (the amount of oxygen in the blood). An alarm started bleeping and I saw the baby's saturation levels were going down rapidly; he was turning blue and was in danger of going into respiratory arrest. I had to react quickly and start to provide emergency oxygen before other people arrived on the scene to help. It was a moment that most student nurses dread, but although frightening it was also very exciting and a good way to test how I would react in an emergency situation. I was relieved that I didn't have time to panic; from my training I knew what to do and acted quickly and automatically.

The most enjoyable experience I have encountered on placement is working alongside a physiotherapist in a burns unit at a specialist children's hospital. The physiotherapist was working with a teenage girl who had been involved in a bad house fire and had lost both her arms and legs, had been in a coma and hadn't walked for eight months. I helped the physiotherapist put on prosthetic legs and helped the patient stand and begin to walk. I was very inspired by how, despite everything, this girl was still positive and fighting to make progress. I learnt that a children's nurse in this role would be involved in wound care, closely monitoring how a patient was coping with trauma both physically and psychologically and ensuring patients regularly did exercises suggested by physiotherapists. I have been inspired to want to be a specialist burns nurse in the future.

My current placement is with a Community Health Visiting Team, working with children's nurses and health visitors, so I can observe both roles. I have been measuring babies' height, weight, length and head circumference, and plotting these on a chart so we can monitor if they are developing normally. This role involves many referrals to other services, such as GPs, dieticians and children's services including child-protection teams. I have had some very useful exposure to other community services and teams, such as school nurses, domestic-violence teams and safeguarding teams, and Children's Centres that help young parents. This has been very useful as there are increasingly more roles for children's nurses in the community. This placement has also provided a chance to provide health-promotion advice and I have learnt the importance of being sensitive to other cultures, beliefs and values when offering advice.

My advice to those wishing to apply for children's nursing is to read articles relating to healthcare and patient care and demonstrate your interest in these topics in your personal statement. Make sure you gain work experience relating to patient care covering a wide age range, not just babies and young children. A children's nurse also works with young adults, parents, families and carers.

Children's nurses within the healthcare system

Traditionally, a common perception has been that sick children are cared for in hospital settings, the place of employment for many children's nurses. Now, however, many children are cared for entirely outside hospital – for many good reasons:

- it enables the child to live in their own home and maintain family and peer relationships
- there is a lower risk of acquiring infection, which is particularly important for those receiving treatment for cancer
- it helps avoid rapidly learned dependence on hospital staff

- it is more cost-effective
- it allows the family to continue to provide personal care, something many people find awkward in hospitals
- it is less stressful for the child, and helps them maintain some control over their care.

With more and more children receiving healthcare outside hospitals, the work locations for children's nurses are also changing, with an increasing number working in private healthcare, social services, the community, schools, children's centres, hospices, charities and a child's own home.

Specialist roles

Specialist roles for children's nurses include caring for children with cancer, asthma or diabetes; neonatal care; nursing children with burns; working with children with special needs; or you could specialise in child protection or caring for children at home.

Intensive care

Children in intensive care often need very intensive support for many months. Children's nurses working in such environments can find themselves drawn into the trauma the family face and, in addition to the 'hands on' care of the child and technical challenges, there are very high levels of responsibility and emotional involvement. In such an environment nurses must also be prepared for the child to not survive, and to support family members and colleagues through the inevitable grief that follows.

Diabetes / epilepsy / asthma

These long-term conditions can affect children at any age. Care is often very successfully managed by the patient/family and/or community nurses. Children with the more common long-term conditions frequently have a specialist children's nurse as their lead health specialist. For example, a paediatric-diabetes nurse specialises in the holistic care of a child with diabetes from infancy through to adolescence, developing, implementing and evaluating programmes of care and providing specialist clinical advice to carers, family, schools and others. Working from a hospital or community base (or both), they will:

- advise on the management of diabetes including diet, medication and complications
- give one-to-one teaching for the child, family and others, particularly promoting safe self-care
- provide counselling
- advise on lifestyle and long-term health issues.

Cancer

We are often reluctant to accept that children get cancer. Survival rates for some cancers have improved dramatically but, even after years of treatment, the outcome may still be death in childhood.

There are a number of roles for children's nurses, including nurses in cancer-care units, where their specialist roles include administration of complex chemotherapy drugs and other treatments, monitoring vital signs, reducing side effects of medication, and strategies to avoid secondary infection, such as nursing the child in isolation facilities. A child may well be known to the hospital nursing team for a year or more, and close relationships can develop; these are often vital for the child and family but can be personally challenging for the nurse.

Children's nurses also work in palliative (end of life) care, both in hospice settings and in the child's own home; these nurses also need psychological skills to support bereaved siblings and families and the ability to make rational professional decisions in the most difficult circumstances.

Mental-health nursing

According to NHS Careers, as many as one in three people are thought to suffer from some sort of mental-health problem. Unlike adult nurses who mainly deal with physical problems that are apparent on the outside, mental-health nurses deal with hidden problems that can only be accessed through communication. The therapeutic relationship is very important; nurses have to use different ways to communicate and engage with people to build trusting relationships. They also use skills to help draw people out and help them explore their own experiences as part of their recovery. They need to be sensitive enough to know when to share aspects of their own life to inspire hope, but also need to maintain professional boundaries. They have to build up a relationship with families and carers so that they can support the client and understand their view of the world in order to be able to help them.

The job can involve working with people with anxiety, depression, stress-related illness, neuroses, psychoses, phobias, post-traumatic-stress disorder, psychological and personality disorders, eating disorders, alcohol and substance-abuse problems, dementia, schizophrenia and paranoia. Patients may have both a learning disability and mental-health issues. The job focuses on promoting recovery or helping clients come to terms with illness and leading a positive life. You must have an awareness of your own mental health and use reflection to understand how your own values and emotions may impact on your own practice. You need to be non-judgemental and able to deal with emotionally charged situations.

In the past people with mental-health problems were cared for only in hospitals and institutions. Since then, there has been much progress in introducing and delivering community care, which aims to support and care for people in their own homes wherever possible, rather than provide care in an institution or residential establishment. A further benefit of community-focused care has been to redefine the relationship between social care and healthcare provision and to encourage partnerships in care between state healthcare providers (e.g. the NHS), local authorities/social services, the private sector and charitable organisations (e.g. Mind).

The job involves:

- having a good understanding of a range of therapies, such as cognitive-behavioural therapy for depression and anxiety
- having in-depth knowledge of mental-health legislation
- using both individual and group interviews to assess clients, produce care plans and set goals
- working with those with critical or acute problems, knowing when to intervene, resolving crises or dealing with a relapse
- working with people who are at risk of suicide and self-harm
- spotting a build-up in tension and diffusing it to avoid violent situations and ensuring that clients remain safe
- raising awareness of mental-health issues and advising other members of the healthcare team
- having in-depth knowledge of medication and the clinical skills to administer drugs and injections, and helping clients make choices about medication, including knowledge of benefits and side effects
- working in multidisciplinary teams in the community to coordinate care of patients.

Case study

Ros Dampier is a second-year mental-health nursing student at De Montfort University. You may find her reasons for choosing mental-health nursing and her experiences on placement helpful to illustrate whether this branch of nursing could be for you.

My current placement is in a treatment and recovery unit for adults with severe, long-standing and complex mental-health conditions. It is a long-stay specialist unit with 19 residents, aged 40 to over 80. I have been assisting residents with personal care, such as washing, dressing and toileting and day-to-day duties such as making beds and helping with mealtimes. I have also been administering medication and giving intramuscular and subcutaneous injections, with direct supervision from my mentor. I spend time talking to residents to assess their needs and to put together a care plan. Residents have both physical and mental-health problems, so I have also been making physical observations, such as temperature and pulse. The role also involves helping with activities for residents to redevelop skills, such as cooking, and trips out to keep them engaged with their community. At shorter-stay units where it is more possible for residents to move on into supported accommodation, there may be more of an emphasis on teaching independent living skills.

Every day there are challenges. When someone opens up to you with something traumatic that has impacted on them in a big way, it is difficult at first to know how to respond – but this is also what is rewarding about the role, that someone trusts you enough to share these feelings and experiences and that you can start to help them deal with them.

I chose mental-health nursing because I have had mental-health problems in the past and wanted to give something back, and because I wanted a job where I could work closely with people, listening to them and talking to them. People often choose to go into this field of nursing because they have experience of mental-health issues, either personally or from a family member. Those who don't can be daunted by stereotypical ideas of people with mental-health issues and be put off applying. My tip would be to get some experience of working with clients with these problems, dispel some of these fears and find out how rewarding it can be. Also, before going to a university selection day, I recommend reading articles relating to mental-health nursing and current issues in nursing in general, in journals such as Nursing Times, Nursing Standard *and* Mental Health Practice, *and to keep up to date with current issues in the news. The NHS Choices website is also useful for easy-to-understand information on health issues.*

TIP

You need to bear in mind that although having mental-health issues yourself can give you an insight into what other sufferers are going through, you need to be well yourself before being able to support and help others and considering applying to mental-health nursing.

Mental-health nurses within the healthcare system

The vast majority of people with mental ill health are cared for in the community, either in their own homes or at clinics and day-care facilities; consequently, the majority of mental-health nurses also work in community settings. Such arrangements allow nurses to offer assessment and therapy, and there are significant advantages to patients and clients:

- it supports independent living, with opportunity for normal family and social relationships
- the patient retains substantial control over the nature and timing of their care.

Mental-health nurses work in:

- prisons/custody centres
- alcohol and/or substance-abuse services
- acute admissions wards
- older persons' mental-health services, e.g. for patients with dementia
- social services, e.g. Child and Adolescent Mental Health Services (CAMHS) or with patients with eating disorders
- secure residential units for adults or children
- voluntary organisations
- residential nursing homes
- people's homes
- hospital outpatients or a specialist unit adjoining a hospital
- community centres and day centres.

Working in such a diversity of settings, especially in the community, mental-health nurses are recognised as lead specialists amongst the diverse multidisciplinary teams supporting their clients.

Specialist roles

Mental-health nurses can specialise in a specific age group, such as children, adults, elderly, or adolescents, or in a particular service, such as alcohol and substance abuse, forensic work, working with offenders, or rehabilitation. The following are some of the specialist areas.

Children/teenagers

Mental-health nurses may work with children with eating disorders or with obsessive-compulsive disorders. Mental-health nurses work with children and young people in their own homes, at school, in community facilities and in hospitals. Quality, trusting relationships, which can take time to establish, are essential in order for nurses to be able to make a detailed assessment and diagnosis prior to planning and delivering therapeutic interventions.

Forensic/secure services

Nurses provide healthcare for people with mental disorders who are offenders or at risk of offending. Services are provided in secure and prison settings. Patients include difficult, dangerous and/or extremely vulnerable people whose behaviour presents a risk to themselves and others. This group of services includes secure services for children and young people. Safe working practices are essential to safeguard patients (both from self-harm and from harm by other patients), staff and the public (to de-escalate potential aggression or disorder).

Pregnancy/childbirth

A woman's mental state can impact on the development of the foetus, the birth of the child, or her family. Depression and anxiety are the most frequent illnesses.

Dementia

According to the Alzheimer's Society, there are 800,000 people in the UK with dementia. Dementia is caused by a brain disease, such as Alzheimer's, or by an injury or a series of mild strokes. It is a progressive disease, often starting with memory problems and leading to difficulties with communication, mood/personality changes and difficulties in coping with daily tasks. As the disease progresses, so independence diminishes. It mostly affects people over 65 but according to the Alzheimer's Society there are over 17,000 people in the UK under the age of 65 who have dementia. Dementia nurses work with families and carers, and collaboratively with other healthcare professionals, to help dementia sufferers develop skills to improve communication, maintain relationships and live as positively as possible.

Learning-disability nursing

In most areas of professional healthcare there is an emphasis on recovery or providing comfort in the end stages of life. For people who have a learning disability, that goal of getting better is not achievable. Instead, learning-disability nurses offer individual support to improve well-being by improving physical and mental health and supporting a person to live an independent and fulfilling life. It can be a demanding and stressful process and one with slow progress; nurses need lots of patience, good communication skills and adaptability, and they may have to deal with challenging behaviour.

What is a learning disability?

According to Mencap (a charity that supports people with learning disabilities), a learning disability is a reduced intellectual ability and difficulty with everyday activities. There are many different types of learning disability, all caused by impaired or disrupted development of the brain, either before birth, or during birth or in early childhood. There is a diverse range of disability levels, with descriptions of mild, moderate, severe or profound-and-multiple-learning disabilities (PMLD) being widely used.

Conditions like Down's syndrome, autism and Asperger's syndrome are not learning disabilities but people with Down's syndrome will all have some degree of learning disability and some people with autism have a learning disability. Therefore, learning-disability nurses regularly work with people with these conditions. They may also work with people with physical conditions, such as cerebral palsy, who in some cases also have a learning disability.

The job involves much interdisciplinary working and in partnership with families and carers. The role involves protecting the rights of those with learning disabilities and challenging negative stereotypes. The role can involve dealing with mild disabilities, such as helping with independent living, and with severe disabilities, where the nursing can focus on providing personal care.

There is also a greater risk of associated physical ill health for people with a learning disability, who may have such conditions as diabetes, epilepsy, impaired vision, defective hearing, speech difficulties and respiratory infections. Learning-disability nurses have to have an understanding of these conditions as well as those of learning disabilities.

Learning Disability Practice magazine (http://learningdisabilitypractice. rcnpublishing.co.uk) may be useful to get a fuller understanding of what learning-disability nursing can entail.

Role of the learning-disability nurse

Learning-disability nurses work with clients of any age, from children to adults. In interdisciplinary and multi-agency teams supporting clients with learning disabilities, learning-disability nurses are frequently the lead practitioner. Since the 1980s there has been progress in introducing and delivering community-care policy, which has changed the whole pattern of care for people with a learning disability and encouraged the delivery of support and care for people in their own homes wherever possible. Significant changes to practices have led to clients receiving care from a partnership of providers, including the NHS, social-care agencies, such as local authorities/social services, housing associations, education centres, and charities, such as Mencap.

Typical day-to-day roles include:

- observing clients, understanding and evaluating behaviour to develop personalised care plans, making home visits and clinic appointments to review progress

- teaching clients the skills to help them live more independently; this might include cleaning teeth, dressing, cooking or making journeys
- leading group sessions on healthy living and behaviour management in supported-living settings
- promoting social inclusion, encouraging and facilitating clients to engage in education, employment, family life and supporting parenting
- promoting rights and choices, advocating on behalf of clients
- developing clients' strengths and abilities
- supporting clients' physical and mental well-being, for example, healthy eating, improving communication skills, helping clients de-escalate stressful/anxious situations
- supporting families of clients and carers, for example, by organising respite care
- using a variety of communication skills to build relationships with clients, adapting information format and presentation, responding to complex behaviours that clients may use as a way of communicating
- liaising with hospital staff on care needs and medication if clients' are admitted to hospital.

Case study

Jessica Potter is a third-year learning-disability nursing student at De Montfort University. You may find it useful to read her reasons for choosing learning-disability nursing, her experiences of being on placement and tips for those who may be considering this branch of nursing.

As part of my BTEC National Diploma in health and social care I did a placement in a day centre for people with learning disabilities. At the end of each day I felt purposeful and that I had made a difference and went home really excited and looking forward to the next day. I also had a placement in a special school and enjoyed working with children with learning disabilities. This confirmed my interest in being a learning-disability nurse.

In the first year of my degree my first placement in learning-disability nursing was in a day centre for people with mild to moderate learning disabilities. This was a good starting point to get a feel for learning-disability nursing.

I followed this by a placement in community nursing and at first was in shock, as the job was so different to what I had expected. It involved making client assessments, relating to vulnerability, mental capacity and risk, meetings and lots of paperwork – with very little obvious clinical nursing. However, as I began to understand the importance of the role – to coordinate support for individuals with a range of learning disabilities – I grew to love it. I also began to understand the meaning of clinical nursing within learning disability which includes screening for mental and physical health as well as therapeutic interventions to help manage a range of physical problems, mental-health problems and challenging behaviour.

I have also had a placement in a 24-hour respite care home for those with more complex needs (where people with learning disabilities can stay to give their carers a break from looking after them) and here I was able to carry out a full range of clinical nursing skills particular to this client group, that included administering medication, PEG feeds (providing nutrition to patients who cannot take in food orally or need nutritional supplements), suctioning (clearing the airway) and management of epilepsy.

My current placement is with the Child and Adolescent Mental Health Services (CAMHS) team. We are working with children with behavioural problems, such as autism, ADHD (attention deficit-hyperactivity disorder) and mental-health problems. All the children have moderate to severe learning disabilities. I have been taking height, weight and blood-pressure measurements in order to review medication. I have learnt a lot about understanding behaviour and working in a multi-professional team. This placement will involve visits to special schools and a children and adolescent mental-health hospital and working with school nurses.

For me, the most challenging placement has been working in a children's hospice – but this has also been the most enjoyable and the type of work I would like to do when I qualify. At first I found being with children with terminal illnesses very upsetting. However, although I became rather attached to one particular child before he died, I found huge satisfaction in making his last days as comfortable as possible. The atmosphere at the hospice was really positive, with a dedicated team of both children's and learning-disability nurses working together to make things as enjoyable as possible for the children.

If you are considering learning-disability nursing, my tip would be to get some relevant work experience and check it is the right course for you. It is very different from adult nursing and quite difficult to get your head around what the job involves unless you see people doing it first-hand.

> *Although you do learn some essential clinical skills, such as administering medication, moving and handling patients, personal care such as bathing, showering and preventing (pressure) sores, giving injections or inserting a feeding tube, the job involves nursing in a much wider context, using communication strategies to promote health and well-being such as therapeutic and non-pharmacological (without the use of drugs) interventions. You have to be passionate about learning-disability nursing because often the importance of the role is underestimated or misunderstood.*

Learning-disability nurses within the healthcare system

Learning-disability nurses often work with clients in their family home or in supported accommodation, a house which has been adapted to become the home of perhaps four clients. They also work in hospital settings with clients who have physical ill health or in secure settings with clients with more complex needs, such as challenging behaviour.

Other places of employment for learning-disability nurses include:

- day centres
- residential care, respite homes, hospices
- prisons/custody centres/young-offender institutions
- schools or special schools, often with residential provision
- supported employment services
- private care homes and clinics.

Specialist roles

Residential home/supported living

Learning-disability nurses in supported-living environments work with clients with mild to moderate learning disabilities who can live independently with some support. The role involves helping them to establish routines such as getting up, dressing and making their own breakfast. You may also work alongside other professionals to help clients to find employment and manage their own money.

In residential homes you may work shifts to support clients with more severe disabilities who require 24-hour care.

Forensic work

Forensic work involves working with clients who have been convicted of a crime but need treatment and support that can't be offered in prison. Learning-disability nurses in this role work in secure hospitals or units for offenders. The role can be demanding, involving the management of challenging behaviour, dealing with ongoing mental-health issues and repeat admissions.

In nursing or care home

In this role you may be caring for people with a combination of learning disabilities, physical disabilities and medical complications. The role can involve building up relationships with clients.

Community nurse

Learning-disability community nurses work in day centres, special schools, adult education, workplaces and people's homes.

Hospital liaison nurse

This role involves being based at a hospital to help learning-disabled clients access health services and to advocate on their behalf. The job also involves training hospital staff to recognise the needs of the learning disabled.

Learning-disability nurses can also choose to work with a specific group of clients, such as those with epilepsy or people with a sensory impairment.

Other specialist roles for nurses

The following are specialist roles open either to all nurses or to those from specific branches of nursing. Information is given on whether these are open to newly qualified nurses or whether you would need specific post-registration experience and further training.

Health visitor

There is currently a drive to recruit more health visitors. Health visitors work with mothers and their babies from the age of around 28 days, taking over from a midwife, and their children up to the age of five. This is a community role, working within a geographical patch, providing physical and developmental checks, parenting advice and supporting mothers with post-natal depression. The job involves support for vulnerable families and involvement in all stages of child-protection cases. There is also a health-promotion role, coordinating health campaigns in partnership with Sure Start Children's Centres. You may be interested in this role if you like working with families and networking with other organisations.

How to become a health visitor

This is open to newly qualified midwives and nurses from all branches of nursing. There is a one-year full-time specialist community public health course (SCPHN/HV), or part-time equivalent. Nurses and midwives are usually seconded by their employer to do this course. See the NHS Careers website for more details, www.nhscareers.nhs.uk.

District nurse

Nurses in this role support patients, families and carers in residential homes, in GP surgeries and at a patient's own home. There is a focus on an educational role: teaching self-care or supporting family members to care for relatives, to allow patients to remain in their own home rather than going into hospital and to minimise readmissions to hospital. District nurses work with patients of all ages, but mostly with the elderly, those recently discharged from hospital, and people who are terminally ill or physically disabled. They mostly work independently, visiting patients in their own homes, sometimes more than once a day, so that relationships can be formed with patients. They also work alongside social services and voluntary agencies.

How to become a district nurse

This is open to newly qualified nurses. There is a 32-week full-time specialist practitioner programme at degree level and part-time routes are also possible. Nurses are usually seconded by their employer.

School nurse

School nurses can be employed by the NHS or directly by a school. The job involves immunisation programmes, developmental screening, giving advice to individuals on health or sex matters, and sex education.

How to become a school nurse

This is open to newly qualified nurses but for some posts experience of working with children, or working in the community, or in health-promotion work may be preferred. You would need to gain the Specialist Practitioner School Nursing/Specialist Community Public Health Nurse qualification available at both degree and master's level. More information is available from the School and Public Health Nurses Association, www.saphna-professionals.org.

Practice nurse

Practice nurses work in GP surgeries, on their own in a small surgery, or in a team in a larger one. The role involves immunisations, family planning and sexual health, health screening, treating minor injuries, including minor surgery, and running vaccination programmes or health-promotion programmes, for example, to help people stop smoking.

Practice nurses can run their own clinics, such as for asthma, diabetes, heart conditions or skin disorders.

How to become a practice nurse

You need to be a registered nurse usually with some post-registration experience. Training programmes are offered by employers on a local basis.

Occupational-health nurse

Occupational-health nurses use their nursing skills in the workplace. They may work in the human-resources department of a company or a university, or in a health-service organisation as an independent practitioner, or for an occupational-health team. The job involves health promotion and health at work, such as first aid and health screening, pre-employment medicals, counselling and support relating to issues such as long-term sickness, workplace health-and-safety legislation, and carrying out risk assessments.

How to become an occupational-health nurse

Post-registration experience is preferred, but is not essential. You will need to gain a Specialist Community Public Health Nursing-Occupational Health Nursing post-registration qualification. See the NMC approved programmes database for courses, www.nmc-uk.org/Approved-Programmes.

Prison nurse

Prison nurses may be employed directly by a prison or by the NHS. They often work partly in the community, partly in prison. The role includes dealing with minor injuries, and mental-health and substance-abuse problems. There is a focus on health-promotion work.

How to become a prison nurse

You need to be a registered adult, mental-health or learning-disability nurse. Specialist training is provided by a prison or the NHS.

Custody nurse practitioner

The Metropolitan Police recruit nurses to care for people in police custody, to make clinical assessments, collect forensic samples and look after the health and welfare of detained persons.

How to become a custody nurse practitioner

A registered adult nurse with experience in A&E, community nursing or the prison service may be preferred. Further training is provided on the job.

Theatre nurse

Theatre nurses work in operating theatres and recovery areas with a range of patients from newborn babies to the elderly. They assist in all stages of patients having an operation: pre-assessment, anaesthesia, surgery and recovery, and answer patients' questions about the benefits and risks of surgical procedures. For this role you need clinical skills, knowledge of specialist equipment and drugs, and specific knowledge to be able to assist an anaesthetist. In the theatre, the work is aseptic (under sterile conditions) and theatre nurses also assist with wound management. They prepare complex machinery, such as lasers and endoscopes (instruments that are used to look inside a person's body), and hand instruments to the surgeon during the operation. After the operation they assess a patient's recovery until they can return to the surgical ward. The role also involves ordering equipment and recording details of the operation.

How to become a theatre nurse

Training is on the job and by completing a part-time in-service course at Diploma in Higher Education, degree or master's level in operating theatre/perioperative care. For more details, see the Association of Perioperative Practice, www.afpp.org.uk.

Neonatal nurse

Neonatal nurses work in specialist units in maternity or children's hospitals or in the community. They work with newborn babies or those who are born sick. The job involves using highly technical equipment and supporting parents who often stay in the hospital to help care for the baby. There is currently a shortage of neonatal nurses, so there are good opportunities to move into this type of work.

How to become a neonatal nurse

Both adult and children's nurses can work in this specialism and would need at least six months' post-registration experience.

Macmillan clinical nurse specialist

It is possible to work with cancer patients for the charity, Macmillan Cancer Support.

How to become a Macmillan clinical nurse specialist

You would need at least five years' post-registration clinical experience, in cancer, palliative care or working with children. Nurses who have worked in the community in an autonomous role are preferred. See www.macmillan.org.uk for more details.

NHS direct nurse adviser

For all branches of nursing there is the chance to work as an NHS direct nurse adviser, answering calls from the public that range from giving advice on health to referring to the emergency services. A high standard of telephone-communication skills is essential.

How to become an NHS direct nurse adviser

You would need post-registration experience: A&E is particularly useful. The training is on the job for 5–12 weeks.

NHS Blood and Transplant (NHSBT) (England and N Wales only), Welsh Blood Service, Scottish National Blood Transfusion Service

Roles in these services involve medical assessments, collecting blood, tissue banking, maintaining the organ-donor register and bone-marrow register, and supervising and training support staff. See www.nhsbtcareers.co.uk for more details.

How to work in NHS Blood and Transplant and in Welsh and Scottish Blood Services

Extensive post-registration experience is needed; experience of critical care or emergency-department nursing may be preferred. See www.nhsbtcareers.co.uk, www.welsh-blood.org.uk or www.scotblood.co.uk for more details.

High-intensity therapist

This option is open both to adult nurses and to mental-health nurses and involves using high-intensity therapeutic interventions, particularly cognitive-behavioural therapy, to support clients with problems related to anxiety and depression. They work in Mental Health Trusts, Primary Care Trusts (PCTs) and charities, and in the independent sector. They may work for the Improving Access to Psychological Therapies Services (IAPT).

How to become a high-intensity therapist

As a registered nurse you would need to do a High Intensity CBT (Cognitive Behavioural Therapy) course: this is a 12-month postgraduate diploma involving both study at university and supervised practice.

In-flight nurse

In-flight nurses work either for the armed forces or for commercial-assistance companies, which provide repatriation services, typically for insurance companies. The work can include repatriating holidaymakers who have become sick on holiday. The role involves assessing a person at a resort, deciding what equipment is needed on the flight, and then making travel arrangements and escorting the person and their family home by commercial airline or air ambulance. Work can also be for overseas companies, government departments and embassies, or for private individuals. In-flight nurses may work freelance or combine office duties in their role. The hours can be long and unpredictable.

How to become an in-flight nurse

You would need about three years' post-registration experience, preferably in adult nursing with experience of acute/critical care. There are also positions for midwives, mental-health nurses and children's nurses who have worked in acute paediatrics. There is a specific training course run by London South Bank University, accredited by the RCN. See www.rcn.org.uk for more details.

Working on a cruise ship

Nurses – normally adult-trained – are employed on cruise ships. They provide patient care to passengers and crew; this can include both outpatient care, such as minor illnesses and accidental injuries, and in-patient care, such as caring for patients with cardiac problems, and medical and surgical emergencies.

How to work on a cruise ship

You would probably need at least three years' post-registration experience, preferably in A&E. Experience in intensive care or cardiac care would also be useful. See www.oceanopportunities.com/medical for further details.

Nurse adviser in the pharmaceutical industry

Nurse advisers are employed by a pharmaceutical company or pharmaceutical organisation to advise NHS staff on best use of pharmaceutical products.

How to become a nurse adviser in the pharmaceutical industry

You would need at least two years' post-registration experience. Some posts may require knowledge of specific diseases.

Career progression

You may decide to focus more on the clinical side of nursing or want to undertake a more managerial post. You may want to get more involved in the education of others or perhaps decide that you like the idea of working in research and helping to develop new treatments and new ways of supporting patients.

Research

You may be interested in a research career, contributing to research studies to collect best evidence to inform clinical decisions and indirectly help patients by improving care delivered. It is possible to receive funding to do a master's degree or a PhD. Internships may also be available to help you prepare for working in a research environment. See the National Institute of Health Research (NIHR) website (www. nihr.ac.uk).

Teaching and assessing

With some post-registration experience you could consider the following roles:

Preceptor

This involves providing support to newly qualified nurses in the first six months of their role.

Mentor

Mentors support student nurses. You can do post-registration courses to prepare for this role.

Practice educator

Practice educators are responsible for teaching and resources in the practice setting and giving guidance to mentors and other health staff who are providing practice placements for students. For this role you may need a postgraduate qualification.

Lecturer

This can involve teaching both pre-registration and post-registration nursing courses at higher-education institutions. Employment is often by universities, where a mixed role of teaching and research is common. Other opportunities are in further education and sixth-form colleges, supporting students undertaking health, social and childcare courses. You would need good interpersonal skills because you would be talking to students individually and also delivering lectures to groups. You could be expected to write articles and publications, so you would need to enjoy writing and presenting your work to colleagues. Nursing lecturers usually have a postgraduate qualification.

Management

There are opportunities to take on supervisory or leadership roles, such as team leader or ward manager, whilst continuing to practise. In senior-management roles you may no longer be a practitioner but focus on management or financial decision making.

Modern matron

Modern matrons have a role which makes them highly visible to patients whilst also being a managerial and clinical professional who is responsible for the management of a group of wards. The role of the modern matron also includes leading and developing the staff team. Other aspects of this post include supporting patients and their families, by being highly visible, and resolving conflicts. Modern matrons also have the responsibility of empowering nurses by supporting them to improve and develop their nursing practice.

Community matron

Community matrons are highly experienced nurses who work independently in the community to organise care plans, mainly for people with long-term conditions or complex conditions. They also act as a point of contact for a caseload of high-intensity users of care services. They can be involved in physical examinations and need diagnostic skills to make decisions, to carry out treatment and prescribe medicines, or to refer to other services. They mostly deal with all ages but some jobs specialise in working with children or the elderly.

Nurse consultant

Very experienced nurses can progress to these positions. Half of their time is spent working directly with patients, the other half being involved in research, education, training and developing nursing practice. They are at the forefront of modernising and improving healthcare services.

Midwifery

To many people, the role of a midwife is to deliver babies. Of course, midwives are certainly key practitioners in assisting women to deliver their babies, but the role is much more than this and includes professional care and support of women both before (antenatal) and after a birth (post-natal). After delivery of the baby, the midwife will continue to be involved in monitoring and assessing the health of both mother and baby, normally for 28 days, although increasingly this role is being per-formed by midwifery care assistants.

Midwives are also the clinical specialists for home births, breastfeeding advice and antenatal screening. They take the lead role in normal preg-nancy and refer to doctors in difficult pregnancies or if there are medical complications during birth. They can work in hospitals and/or the com-munity. The role involves supporting an increasing number of women of ethnic diversity, including those where English isn't their first language.

What do midwives do?

- Diagnosing pregnancy, making assessments, history taking, physi-cal examinations, monitoring condition of the foetus, screening and blood tests, identification of any complications
- Providing health education and parenting advice for the mother, her partner and perhaps other family members, including daily care of baby, child development and promoting breastfeeding
- Providing advice and support following events such as miscarriage, termination of pregnancy, stillbirth, birth abnormality, neonatal death and post-natal depression
- Prescribing and administering medication, especially pain relief
- Managing labour and childbirth
- listening to women and enabling them to make informed choices about the birth and care of their baby, including birth plans, advice on where to have a baby, plans for feeding, post-natal support and preparation for parenthood
- negotiating with health professionals about birth plans
- Emergency procedures, including resuscitation of mother and baby, removal of placenta
- Examining baby after birth and taking action if needed
- Care for those who have had a Caesarean section
- Examining and caring for babies with low birth weight, birth defects, pre-term babies or those with disabilities
- Health-promotion work in the community.

Case study

Amanda Mallett is a recently qualified midwife. Her experiences may help you decide whether midwifery is for you.

Before having time off to have her children, Amanda had previously worked in office jobs and knew that she wanted to retrain for a career where she could work in a very different environment. With some encouragement from friends she decided on midwifery. As she hadn't studied for many years she was advised that an Access to Higher Education Diploma would be the most suitable route to a midwifery degree. She found the course particularly useful for re-establishing skills that she was rusty in, such as writing essays and taking exams. The course also helped her develop research and presentation skills, essential to undertake a university degree. The Access course modules she took were specific to going on to a nursing or midwifery degree and covered subjects such as anatomy and physiology. These topics also featured in the first year of her course, so she felt she had had a head start.

Alongside her Access course she got some work experience as a volunteer on a hospital maternity ward. The tasks were administrative rather than clinical, but she did get an insight into what midwives do. Through a friend, she also managed to shadow a midwife.

She was successful in getting a place on a midwifery degree and later in getting a job as a midwife in the hospital local to the course where she had done many of her placements.

Initially the job involved spending two-week blocks in the antenatal ward, post-natal ward and the delivery suite. The antenatal ward involves working with women who have come into hospital because they have problems with pregnancy, such as hyperemesis gravidarum (severe sickness leading to dehydration) or need to be induced because they have diabetes or have gone beyond their due date. Post-natal work involves looking after mother and baby, particularly first-time mums who need help with breastfeeding. The midwife has an educational role to provide information and advice. It can also involve looking after women who have had a Caesarean section or an instrumental delivery, where post-operative care is needed. On the delivery suite the work can involve women in early labour or later stages of labour and includes triage work: midwife-led assessments with referral to a doctor if needed.

She works shifts which can include nights, bank holidays, even Christmas Day, to ensure 24-hour care. She would advise anyone interested in midwifery to get a job which gives them a taste of shift work before deciding on this career. She pointed out that until you are regularly doing shift work you don't fully appreciate how it can impact on daily life, particularly if you have children.

She thinks the most important qualities a midwife needs are a desire to care for people and to be a good communicator. In particular, verbal-communication skills are needed to work with a whole range of people on different levels, from patients and their families, to care assistants to doctors.

The biggest challenge of the job for Amanda is when non-anticipated complications suddenly arise during labour and childbirth. However, in her first few months of the job she has been in awe of how smoothly the healthcare team swings into action; everyone is totally clear about what they need to do and she knows this level of confidence will come with time and experience. She now appreciates why she was advised to spend at least a year being hospital-based before considering working in the community, because you are supported by a team in these emergency situations, rather than working on your own.

In the future she would like to be a community midwife as she is attracted to the continuity of care that is possible in this role, particularly with respect to women who opt for home births. You can support the whole process, from first meeting a woman, seeing them through the cycle of pregnancy, looking after them in labour, delivering their baby and helping mum and baby through home visits, until the baby is 28 days old, when responsibility is handed over to a health visitor. This can be a very autonomous role; for women where pregnancy is straightforward the midwife will have sole care without involving a doctor.

Amanda's tip would be to work as a maternity care assistant. She feels that this is a very good preparation for applying to a midwifery degree as it shows commitment to this type of work and gives you a real insight into some aspects of the work of a midwife, such as making observational checks, breastfeeding support and working shifts. She would also advise reading midwifery journals, such as *Midwives* magazine, to demonstrate that you have knowledge of current midwifery issues.

Where midwives work

- Midwives work in NHS or private hospitals, antenatal and post-natal wards and in labour ward/delivery suite, neonatal units. Antenatal care may involve women experiencing complications such as pre-eclampsia, a condition potentially harmful (even fatal) to both mother and baby. Post-natal care includes care of women (and their babies) where birth has been difficult or traumatic, for example, where surgical repair or Caesarean section has been necessary.
- Midwives work in the community where they offer antenatal and post-natal care for women in their own homes, GP surgeries, health clinics, and in children's centres. They support home births. Community midwives are most commonly employed by the NHS, although a smaller number work independently.

 • Birth centres are midwife-led units (either NHS or private). They can be based either in a hospital or separate from it.

Specialist roles for midwives

Midwives can work in a variety of settings and many remain in hospitals whilst others move into the community and work in GP practices, for charities and in children's centres. Many jobs are also integrated, which means that post holders spend time working in the community and in a hospital setting.

You may also wish to focus on a particular aspect of midwifery and develop your expertise in a specific clinical area. Midwives can specialise in areas such as public health, parenting education, ultrasound and foetal medicine.

Advanced-practitioner posts

There are advanced-practitioner posts, such as lead midwife for breast-feeding, where you would be expected to promote breastfeeding within the maternity unit to midwives, allied health professionals and to the wider community. You would have developmental responsibilities and be expected to devise and implement new ways of working. You would also be expected to collect, analyse and disseminate data to show how your area of responsibility is developing. There would be a training element to your work: you would be teaching staff who are working with mothers. Alongside these duties, you would continue to practise as a midwife and act as a role model for new and experienced staff.

Advanced-practitioner posts, such as this, are suitable for anyone who is a good clinician and a confident communicator who enjoys working with a wide variety of people, from women and their families to professionals in healthcare and related services. It is the type of role that needs someone who also has strong organisational and project-development skills.

Management roles

You may enjoy organising, planning and developing systems and staff. If this is you, you might consider a managerial post such as a midwifery team leader in a labour or post-natal ward. Such a post would include being responsible for the day-to-day management of the midwifery services in your ward. You would lead the team, organise workloads and ensure that care is effectively delivered with the resources available. Staff recruitment and development would also be part of your remit. You would continue to practise as a midwife and act as a professional lead in your ward, providing advice to other midwives and health professionals when required. It may be the type of post that would suit you if you enjoy developing processes and ensuring that services are delivered to a high standard.

Teaching and research

Returning to higher education as a lecturer is another role that experienced midwives can access. If you enjoy learning, you can continue to enhance your education by studying for a master's degree and then for a PhD. If you enjoy research and teaching, career opportunities exist as lecturers and subsequently professors of midwifery in universities. Such careers would immerse you in the clinical development and education of new midwives. This would involve one-to-one support, running tutorials and lectures. You would also be expected to conduct research on areas of midwifery in which you had a professional interest.

Further training

Most nurses and midwives undertake additional training to extend their skills and knowledge, to progress or specialise.

Anyone who has completed a diploma course in nursing may be able to top up their qualification to a degree through part-time study whilst in nursing employment. This is not a requirement for practice but may be beneficial for career development or necessary to access higher-level courses.

A wide range of postgraduate courses are available at universities for qualified nurses and midwives who wish to enhance their skills or training. For those wanting to expand their professional knowledge, master's degree courses and postgraduate diplomas are available in subjects such as:

- specialist community-health nursing – in a range of specialist areas, such as school nursing, occupational-health nursing
- community nursing practice – including prescribing medicines qualifications
- advanced nursing practice – includes leadership skills, advanced decision making, evidence-based practice
- midwifery and women's health
- advanced midwifery practice.

Some nurses and midwives decide that they want to research in far greater depth a specific area of clinical interest and subsequently opt to study a PhD.

Working overseas

Qualified nurses and midwives are in demand to work overseas on long-term development projects to train or support local health staff to develop skills and services. An example of this would be preventive work, treatment and support for people with HIV and AIDS in Africa. Nurses and midwives are also needed on shorter-term projects to provide emergency care after conflict or a natural disaster.

Nurses with experience of paediatrics, emergency care, theatre nursing or public-health work in the community are preferred. You would need at least two years' experience, although upwards of five years' experience is preferred. Experienced mental-health nurses are also needed to support people after conflict or a natural disaster.

The role of working overseas can involve giving advice on nutrition, immunisation, assessing refugees or assisting traditional birth attendants. Supervisory skills are needed as are the flexibility and resourcefulness to adapt local equipment and resources. The job may involve training nurses and midwives, including classroom teaching. It is vital to be able to maintain professionalism but also to think quickly, rationally and with cultural sensitivity.

Resources are often extremely limited (e.g. intermittent electricity); conditions and equipment are often basic: lack of medicines, lack of clean/running water or difficulty in maintaining a clean environment. The range of needs encountered will include many of those experienced by patients in the UK/Europe together with many more, including local/tropical disease and trauma/emergency situations that at home would be dealt with by a much more comprehensive team.

The work is usually voluntary or with a low basic pay rate or cost-of-living allowance. You would need to bear in mind that in order to maintain your NMC registration, you would have to keep up with your continuing professional development (CPD) whilst abroad.

It is possible to work for large organisations such as Médecins sans Frontières or VSO or smaller organisations. See the Royal College of Nursing guide, 'Working with Humanitarian Organisations' (2010), available to download from www.rcn.org.uk, for more information.

The armed forces

The British Army, Royal Navy and RAF employ registered adult and mental-health nurses. A common misconception is that nursing in the military is all about front-line duties, but this is only one of the many locations of deployment.

Adult nurses may find themselves working in any of a particularly broad range of locations, in environments that may be unpredictable, intense and time-pressured, as patient assessment and management decisions need to be made rapidly.

Mental-health nurses are likely to encounter clients with mental-health problems exacerbated by traumatic or upsetting experiences, especially amongst those in front-line combatant roles. Problems such as post-traumatic-stress disorder may be encountered more frequently.

Advanced and specialist job roles are also available for those interested in specialising in the care of patients with specific illnesses. Nurses undertaking these roles are required to have further specialist knowledge and skills in specific clinical areas. They may run their own clinics.

Army

Army nurses may work in field hospitals, dealing with casualties and victims of trauma but equally in medical regiments, Ministry of Defence (MOD) hospital units in the UK, in management, recruitment and personnel, and also in education and training. Progression routes include nurses being able to work up to nursing-officer posts, which involve leading and developing a team of nurses, and planning and delivering nursing care. See www.army.mod.uk for further information.

Navy

Nurses in the navy can work both on shore and at sea, including in MOD hospital units, and provide medical support to Royal Navy and Royal Marines both in the UK and around the world. They can take courses in intensive care, operating theatres, emergency medicine, orthopaedics, primary care and mental health. See www.royalnavy.mod.uk/careers for further information.

RAF

The RAF employs adult nurses to look after the health and fitness of aircrew, ground crew and support staff; nurses can be based in medical centres on RAF stations in the UK and overseas or at MOD hospital units. They may also be deployed to field hospitals or be involved in projects to evacuate casualties from overseas to hospitals in the UK. See www.raf.mod.uk/careers for further details.

Associated careers

The following are associated roles that you may wish to consider to help you decide whether studying nursing or midwifery is the most appropriate route for you.

Nursery nurse

Despite the title, nursery nurses work predominantly in childcare rather than having a healthcare role. They assist babies and young children with play, learning, social development and personal care in local-authority or private nurseries, schools and in private homes (as nannies).

Healthcare assistant (sometimes known as nursing auxiliary or support worker)

Healthcare assistants work alongside and support other health professionals, such as nurses, in hospitals or community settings. There are many variations to the role but the focus is on personal care and patient comfort. Some healthcare assistants undertake training to extend their role or to specialise – this can sometimes be a route into professional nursing or midwifery.

Carer

A carer is someone who provides help and support to a partner, family or friends without being paid. Carers give assistance to people who need additional help because of age, illness or disability.

Health visitor

Health visitors are qualified nurses or midwives who have completed further specialist training. The role of a health visitor is to work as a lead member of the primary healthcare team. They are concerned with promoting health and well-being in the community. Most of the work involves supporting families and pre-school children, including babies from about 28 days old.

Midwifery care assistant

Midwifery care assistants work alongside and support midwives and are taking on increasing responsibility for post-natal care. Working as a midwifery care assistant can provide excellent work experience for applying to a midwifery degree.

12 | Further information

Nursing and midwifery professional organisations

Nursing and Midwifery Council
23 Portland Place
London W1B 1PZ
Tel: 020 7637 7181 (general enquiries)
Tel: 020 7333 9333 (registration enquiries)
www.nmc-uk.org

Royal College of Midwives
15 Mansfield Street
London W1G 9NH
Tel: 020 7312 3535
www.rcm.org.uk

Royal College of Nursing
20 Cavendish Square
London W1G 0RN
Tel: 020 7409 3333
www.rcn.org.uk

Journals/magazines

Learning Disability Practice
http://learningdisabilitypractice.rcnpublishing.co.uk

Mental Health Practice
http://mentalhealthpractice.rcnpublishing.co.uk

Midwives
www.rcm.org.uk/midwives

Nursing Children and Young People
http://nursingchildrenandyoungpeople.rcnpublishing.co.uk

Nursing Standard
http://nursingstandard.rcnpublishing.co.uk

Nursing Times
www.nursingtimes.net

Study and training

UCAS
Customer Contact Centre
UCAS, PO Box 28
Cheltenham GL52 3LZ
Tel: 0871 468 0468 (customer service unit)
www.ucas.com (search and apply for pre-registration nursing and midwifery courses)

UKPass
www.ukpass.ac.uk (search and apply for postgraduate courses)

www.studentmidwife.net

Careers

Armed forces careers
Army: www.army.mod.uk/careers
Royal Navy: www.royalnavy.mod.uk/careers
Royal Air Force: www.raf.mod.uk/careers

Learning-disability nursing
www.learningdisabilitynurse.com

NHS Careers
Tel: 0345 606 0655 (careers helpline)
www.nhscareers.nhs.uk
www.stepintothenhs.nhs.uk
www.whatcanidowithmydegree.nhs.uk (careers in the NHS for graduates)
www.jobs.nhs.uk

Prospects
(graduate careers website and information on postgraduate study)
www.prospects.ac.uk

Funding

HSC Nursing and Midwifery Bursary (Northern Ireland)
Tel: 028 9053 5575
www.nursingandmidwiferycareersni.com

NHS Student Bursaries (England)
Hesketh House
200–220 Broadway
Fleetwood FY7 8SS
Tel: 0845 358 6655
www.nhsbsa.nhs.uk/students

NHS Wales Student Awards Unit
Tel: 02920 196167
www.wales.nhs.uk/sitesplus/829/page/36092

Student Awards Agency for Scotland (SAAS)
Tel: 0300 555 0505
www.saas.gov.uk

Student Finance England
Tel: 0845 300 5090
www.sfengland.slc.co.uk

Student Finance Wales
Tel: 0845 602 8845
www.studentfinancewales.co.uk

Other useful websites

BBC News
www.bbc.co.uk/news/health

Department of Health
www.dh.gov.uk

Disclosure and Barring Service (DBS) (formerly CRB)
Tel: 0870 909 0811
www.gov.uk/crb-criminal-records-bureau-check

Disclosure Scotland
Tel: 0870 609 6006
www.disclosurescotland.co.uk

NHS
www.nhs.uk (England)
www.show.scot.nhs.uk (Scotland)
www.wales.nhs.uk (Wales)
www.n-i.nhs.uk (Northern Ireland)

Glossary

Acute care
Short-term hospital treatment for a severe injury or illness or urgent medical condition. It can refer to any area of nursing practice, including adult (e.g. people with pneumonia – acute medical care, appendicitis – acute surgical care); children's (e.g. a child dehydrated from diarrhoea, a child with a burn injury); mental health (e.g. a person with psychosis or paranoia).

Ambulatory care
Medical care that does not require an overnight stay in a hospital, such as that provided on an outpatient basis.

Anaesthetic
A drug that temporarily reduces or takes away sensation, so that otherwise painful procedures or surgery can be performed. A local anaesthetic numbs one part of the body, such as a hand or leg. A general anaesthetic artificially induces a controlled loss of consciousness (being 'put to sleep'), most commonly so that a person is pain-free and not aware of a surgical procedure.

Anatomy
The study of the structure of the body, from cellular to skeletal.

Antenatal
The care of pregnant women prior to the birth of the baby – in other words, up to the time of labour and delivery.

Aseptic
A procedure that is performed under sterile conditions, to minimise exposure to germs.

Bipolar disorder
Bipolar disorder, previously known as manic depression, is a condition that affects a person's moods, which can swing from one extreme to the other, from 'high' (mania) to 'low' (depression), with varying degrees of severity. It is a long-term mental-health condition.

Caesarean section
Surgery to deliver a baby, where the baby is taken out through the mother's abdomen. Caesareans can be emergency (performed during labour due to necessity) or can be planned or elective (performed prior to labour for medical reasons or if requested by a patient).

Cannulation

A cannula is a fine plastic tube. Of the many diverse types and uses, by far the most common is a venous cannula, inserted into a vein to deliver fluid or drugs or to take blood samples. Cannulation (putting the cannula in) is a skill used by midwives and also by nurses in many settings.

Cardiovascular

Relating to the circulatory system, which comprises the heart and blood vessels.

Carer

Provides help and support to a partner, family or friends without being paid.

Clinical simulation suites

Universities' departments set up to mirror hospital, community or home settings to enable students to practise real-life clinical skills and procedures in safe and supervised conditions. Computerised dummies, called 'sim men', are used to create a realistic experience; these are models which breathe and talk and can simulate conditions such as cardiac arrest or falling blood pressure. The rooms also include equipment such as electric beds, moving and handling equipment, and monitoring equipment.

Clinical skills

Procedures used to care for and treat patients.

Cognitive-behavioural therapy

A therapy aimed at helping the patient manage their problems in a more positive way by changing the way they think (cognitive) and behave.

Continuing professional development (CPD)

Learning and development activities to ensure that professionals keep their knowledge and skills up to date in order to continue to be competent to practise safely. CPD is necessary for nurses to remain on the NMC register to practise as a nurse or midwife.

COPD (chronic obstructive pulmonary disease)

One of the most common respiratory conditions in the UK, COPD describes a number of lung diseases including chronic bronchitis, emphysema and chronic obstructive airways disease. People with COPD have difficulties in breathing, primarily due to the narrowing of their airways. The main cause of COPD is smoking.

Dementia

Dementia is usually caused by a brain disease, such as Alzheimer's. It is progressive, often starting with memory problems, leading to difficulties with communication, mood changes and difficulties in coping with daily tasks.

Depot injection
Slow-release medication given to regulate a person's behaviour, used by mental-health or learning-disability nurses.

Domiciliary care
Care given in a person's home to enable them to live independently.

Endoscope
An instrument used to see inside the body. It is usually a long thin tube with a light and camera on the end.

Evidence-based practice
To deliver care based on the best available evidence or practice. This means keeping up to date with developments in research and practice.

Forensic nursing
Working with offenders or those at risk of offending.

HDU (high-dependency unit)
These can be found in hospitals supporting adults or children with either physical or mental ill health. HDUs are often described as a 'step-up' or 'step-down' unit – between a general ward and an intensive-care or critical-care unit. People in an HDU generally need frequent assessment and more concentrated care than is typical of a general ward, but without the life-support equipment of intensive care. HDUs have a high staff–patient ratio.

Holistic care
Universally promoted in nursing and midwifery, holistic care recognises that all aspects of a person should be considered in order to care for the person as a whole. This means carefully taking into account not just immediate physical or mental-health needs, but also all psychological, environmental and spiritual needs.

Hospital Trusts
An organisation that provides hospital services, either NHS or independent. An NHS Hospital Trust, also known as an acute trust, is an NHS Trust that provides hospital services either from one hospital or from a group of hospitals in a specific geographical area.

Injections
Used to give small volumes of fluid to a patient, almost always solutions of drugs. There are many types of injection: intravenous (into a vein); intramuscular (into a muscle); subcutaneous (just under the skin); and intradermal (into the skin).

Instrumental delivery
Using instruments such as forceps or a ventouse vacuum device to assist the delivery of a baby.

Intensive care/critical care

Intensive-care units (ICUs) are specialist hospital wards to provide intensive treatment and monitoring for people who are critically ill or in an unstable position, after surgery, an accident or after severe illness. Patients need constant medical attention and support to keep their body functioning. They may be unable to breathe on their own or have multiple-organ failure.

Intrapartum

The period of childbirth or delivery.

Long-term condition

A health condition that is serious but not life-threatening but which needs continuing care.

Mentoring

Two (or more) people working together to further learning and development of skills. Mentoring is a key part of nursing and midwifery courses where on each placement the student is closely supported by a mentor, who is a trained and experienced practitioner.

MRSA

A bacterial infection that is resistant to a number of antibiotics and can lead to life-threatening infections.

Multidisciplinary working

Multidisciplinary working involves staff from several different professional backgrounds, with different areas of expertise, working together. It can also be called partnership working, multi-professional working or collaborative working. Nurses in the community commonly work in this way, for example, mental-health nurses within community mental-health teams (CMHT) or within child and adolescent mental-health services (CAMHS).

Neonatal

Relating to newborn babies up to a few weeks of age.

Neurological

Illnesses or treatments connected to the nervous system: the brain, spinal cord or nerves.

OSCE (objective structured clinical examination)

Practical examinations used to test clinical skills and competence that form part of pre-registration nursing and midwifery training. A student is given a scenario relating to an individual patient, has to make an observation, carry out an assessment and then suggest how to treat, backing this up with evidence. This may take place in a simulation suite using a 'sim man', a mannequin that breathes and talks and mimics human reactions.

Palliative care

Any healthcare intended to reduce the severity of symptoms (e.g. pain) rather than providing a cure or slowing progression of a disease.

Palliative care aims to minimise suffering and improve quality of life rather than routinely planning to extend life as long as possible. Palliative care is provided in hospices for those with a terminal illness (where a cure is no longer possible) or for those near the end of their life.

PEG (percutaneous endoscopic gastronomy) feed
Providing nutrition to a patient who cannot take food orally or who needs nutritional supplements, by inserting a feeding tube.

Perinatal
The time immediately before and/or after birth.

Pharmacology
The study of drugs, their effects on the body and their administration.

Physiology
The study of how the body functions, for example, processes such as digestion, blood flow and pain. It is important for nurses and midwives to have a good understanding of physiology, as it is closely linked to clinical decisions concerned with blood pressure, wound healing, pain management etc.

Post-natal
The period immediately after the birth of the baby until the child is about one month old.

Post-registration courses
Career-development courses for qualified and registered nurses and midwives.

Post-registration education and practice (PREP) standards
To maintain registration with the NMC, nurses and midwives need to meet certain standards, called PREP. These involve completing a specific number of practice hours and learning activities prior to a review of their registration, to ensure that they are still competent to practise.

Preceptorship
The initial probationary period of a nursing or midwifery job, usually 6 to 12 months, where nurses and midwives are given support and supervision to enable transition into the position and to ensure that they are practising competently and safely.

Primary care
Care provided in the community, such as at GP surgeries, at clinics, and by dentists and pharmacists, and is usually the first point of contact for patients in the NHS.

Primary-care trusts (PCTs)
Primary-care trusts (there are currently 151 in England) manage the services provided by doctors, dentists, opticians and pharmacists. Primary-care services are usually the first point of contact for patients when

they have a health problem. PCTs work with local authorities and other agencies to provide health and social-care services.

Resuscitation
An emergency procedure for people whose heart has stopped (cardiac arrest – mostly adults) or who have stopped breathing (respiratory arrest – adults or children) or both. CPR is the abbreviation for cardio-pulmonary resuscitation, the process of compressing the chest and artificially ventilating (inflating) the lungs.

Safeguarding
Ensuring the safety and promoting the welfare of children and vulnerable adults. Nurses and midwives have a duty to be alert to signs of maltreatment that may impair health or development.

Service user
A receiver of health or care services, a term used most often in mental-health care.

Substance abuse
Harmful use of addictive substances, such as alcohol and drugs.

Suctioning
Using a device, usually an electrically operated vacuum pump, to clear the airways of blood, saliva or vomit so that a patient can breathe.

Therapeutic interventions
General term used to describe interactions with patients to improve health and well-being. This can include specific therapies, such as cognitive-behavioural therapy.

Transferable skills
Skills gained in one setting that can be used in a number of different settings, such as communication skills, organisational skills and team-working.